PRAISE FOR *VEGAN FOR LIFE*

"The vegan revolution is upon us! *Vegan for Life* is an essential handbook for understanding all of the ins and outs of this increasingly popular lifestyle choice."

> —Mark Reinfeld, coauthor of *The 30-Minute Vegan*, *The 30-Minute Vegan's Taste of the East*, *The Idiot's Guide to Eating Raw*, and *Vegan Fusion World Cuisine*

"In a clear and concise manner, vegan nutritionists Jack and Virginia spell out what it really means to be healthy. Reading this well presented, fact-based book about your well-being and the well-being of our planet, you'll be equipped with all the necessary tools to achieve your own personal best in health."

> —Robert Cheeke, best-selling author of *Vegan Bodybuilding & Fitness*

"*Vegan For Life* shows not only the adequacy and benefits of a vegan diet, but the steps to make the transition and do it right! It's the book I recommend to all of my clients."

> —Matt Ruscigno, MPH, RD

VEGAN FOR LIFE

VEGAN FOR LIFE

Everything You Need to
Know to Be Healthy and Fit
on a Plant-Based Diet

Jack Norris, RD
Virginia Messina, MPH, RD

Da Capo
∞
LIFE
LONG

A Member of the Perseus Books Group

Designed by Trish Wilkinson
Set in 11.5 point Goudy Old Style

Cataloging-in-Publication data for this book is available from the Library of Congress.

First Da Capo Press edition 2011
ISBN: 978-0-7382-1493-1
E-book ISBN: 978-0-7382-1497-9

Published by Da Capo Press
A Member of the Perseus Books Group
www.dacapopress.com

Note: The information in this book is true and complete to the best of our knowledge. This book is intended only as an informative guide for those wishing to know more about health issues. In no way is this book intended to replace, countermand, or conflict with the advice given to you by your own physician. The ultimate decision concerning care should be made between you and your doctor. We strongly recommend you follow his or her advice. Information in this book is general and is offered with no guarantees on the part of the authors or Da Capo Press. The authors and publisher disclaim all liability in connection with the use of this book.

Da Capo Press books are available at special discounts for bulk purchases in the U.S. by corporations, institutions, and other organizations. For more information, please contact the Special Markets Department at the Perseus Books Group, 2300 Chestnut Street, Suite 200, Philadelphia, PA, 19103, or call (800) 810-4145, ext. 5000, or e-mail special.markets@perseusbooks.com.

10 9 8 7 6 5 4 3 2

To all farmed animals,
and to those who work to end their suffering.

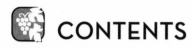 CONTENTS

INTRODUCTION
Going Vegan for Life

A vegan diet is the world's most simple solution to a host of complex problems.

For almost all of human history, people ate whatever they could get their hands on; availability, habit, and taste preferences were the factors that drove food choices. That changed a mere century or so ago, when the new science of nutrition revealed that food was more than just something to eat—it was part of an approach to optimal health.

But in the past few decades, we've come to understand that what we eat has more far-reaching effects. Not just on our health but on the lives of the animals who share this planet with us and on the very future of the planet itself. Our current food system supports a growing health crisis in America, a worrisome loss of global resources, and some of the worst cruelty to animals imaginable. Today, there are a lot of good reasons to embrace a vegan diet.

Going vegan is easy and fun. But without a doubt, there is a little bit of a learning curve. That's why we wrote this book—to provide both newcomers and more seasoned vegans with solid information that will keep your diet healthy and practical.

As dietitians and animal advocates, we are unapologetically pro-vegan, and we want to help as many people as possible take steps toward an animal-free diet. That means that we want you to have the best nutrition advice possible, because a vegan diet isn't a realistic choice if you aren't meeting your nutrient needs or eating in a way that supports optimal health. We'll give you all of the basic nutrition information—the absolutely essential facts that you need to safeguard your health while moving toward a vegan diet. We've also provided plenty of practical tips and tools to make the transition easy.

For those who are new to veganism, we hope the information in this book will reassure you that a vegan diet is safe and healthy. But we think that longtime vegans will find plenty of useful information here as well. We're going to sort through myths that have caused some vegans to make less-than-optimal food choices and give you ideas on how to make your vegan diet even healthier.

And if you are just dipping your toe in the water, that's fine. Use the information here to start a transition, because even reducing the amounts of animal foods in your diet makes a big difference.

GOING VEGAN IS EASIER THAN EVER

Veganism may seem like something new and unusual, but it's a concept that has been around for awhile. In 1944, just after the end of World War II, a small group of British vegetarians added the word "vegan" to our language. It was derived from the first three and last two letters of the word "vegetarian" because, they said, "Veganism starts with vegetarianism and carries it through to its logical conclusion."

It was not an easy time to be a vegan, especially in England. Postwar food shortages made any kind of special diet difficult. The science of nutrition was young, and some nutrients of specific concern to vegans hadn't even been identified yet. Nobody had ever heard of veganism, so it stands to reason that resources like cookbooks were nonexistent.

The change we're seeing sixty-five years later would have astounded those early pioneers. In fact, they astound some of us who have been vegan for a mere twenty years. Not only do we have hundreds of vegan cookbooks, but we also have cookbooks devoted to vegan baking, holiday celebrations, meals for kids, and backyard barbecues. Nearly every grocery store in America carries soymilk, veggie hotdogs, and dairy-free ice cream. And if you can't find what you want in your local market, there are online vegan grocery stores to fill almost every need.

All of these changes conspire to make vegan eating easier and more appealing than you may have ever imagined. Vegans still eat beans and rice, but they also eat pasta with artichoke pesto, tempeh roasted in apricot barbecue sauce, hot fudge sundaes, and veggie cheeseburgers. With better food, more information, and a growing appreciation of the health benefits of plant foods, the world is becoming more vegan friendly.

WHY VEGAN?

Since 1950, profound changes have taken place on farms, driven by efforts to cut costs and produce cheap meat, milk, and eggs. The changes have given birth to factory farms, where animals are crammed into sheds and cages with virtually no room to move. Modern farming ignores the basic instinctual needs and welfare of individual animals. Many die before they ever make it to the slaughterhouse from disease or injury or because they couldn't access food or water. Conditions at slaughterhouses are deplorable and cruel as well. Today's farm is less likely to be a friendly family enterprise and more likely to be a factory where efficiency takes precedence over respectful treatment of animals. The plain and simple—and uncomfortable—fact is that production of animal foods (even dairy and eggs) contributes to animal suffering.

Thanks to the work of animal-rights organizations, more people are becoming aware of these abuses. One answer for many has been to seek out foods from animals who were raised more humanely. Many products that boast "humanely produced" type labels come from animals who lived under somewhat better circumstances, but often the differences are negligible. And all of these animals usually go to the same slaughterhouses. Likewise, the term "organic" doesn't translate to "humanely produced." A large percentage of organic animal foods come from animals who were raised on factory farms.

Any truly meaningful welfare improvements can take place only on very small farms where every phase of the animal's life (and death) is monitored. But that's a costly and inefficient way to produce animal foods. Even if people could afford them, there isn't enough land for farms of this type to feed the American population.

In Chapter 16, we'll look at these issues in more depth. It's not easy to read about the lives of these animals, but if you are wondering whether a vegan diet is the right choice for you, we think that the information will provide some perspectives on food choices. Whether you are concerned about the suffering of factory-farmed animals or embrace the belief that animals should never be used by humans, a vegan diet is an effective and meaningful way to put these beliefs into practice.

Meat, dairy, and egg production is also wasteful and harmful to the environment. Land that is used to raise food for billions of farm animals could grow food for direct human consumption, saving forests, water, and fossil fuels. A reduced dependence on animal foods is a significant step toward making your carbon footprint smaller.

Finally, those who opt for a plant-based diet are likely to enjoy personal benefits as well. Vegans have lower cholesterol and less hypertension and are less likely to develop diabetes. And vegan diets have been used as part of successful programs for treating chronic disease. We'll look at those issues in Chapter 13.

ARE VEGAN DIETS SAFE?

According to the American Dietetic Association, vegan diets are safe for all stages of the life cycle as long as they are well planned.[1] The "well-planned" caveat has been a source of annoyance among vegan dietitians for nearly two decades. Any diet, vegan or not, has to be well-planned. Those who consume animal products don't automatically meet all nutrient needs and can fall short on fiber and other compounds that are abundant in vegan diets. Likewise, vegan diets require more attention to some nutrients like vitamin B_{12} and iron.

The point is that everyone, no matter what type of diet they eat, needs a little nutrition know-how. But yes, vegan diets can—and do—support optimal health throughout the life cycle. Many of the negative stories about vegans, especially children, who suffer from nutrient deficiencies are actually due to very restrictive types of vegan diets such as macrobiotic or raw foods.

A vegan diet isn't difficult; it's just a different way of meeting nutrient needs. This book is a guide to vegan nutrition and meal planning at all stages of the life cycle as well as for those who wish to adopt a vegan diet to reduce their risk for chronic disease. We've provided steps that translate nutrition information into real food choices and realistic menus for everyone.

Going vegan for life is a choice that has win-win written all over it. It respects the lives of animals and represents a refusal to contribute to their suffering. Many people feel a sense of relief when they start taking steps toward veganism because it reflects how they feel about animals. A plant-based menu is also broadening and will introduce you to new foods and menus; it's very likely to make your diet more interesting, not less. And depending on what your diet is like right now, making the move toward veganism is very likely to improve your health.

This book is for everyone who wants to reap these benefits and is ready to get started on the path to compassionate and healthy eating.

A Few Definitions

Omnivore
In this book, we use the terms "omnivore" and "meat-eater" to describe anyone who chooses to include meat and other animal foods in his or her diet. So, an omnivore is someone who eats plants, meat, dairy foods, and eggs.

Plant-based diets
Some omnivores eat a plant-based diet. That is, they eat meat, dairy, and eggs, but they emphasize plant foods in their meals, usually for health reasons. The terms "flexitarian" and "semi-vegetarian" are also used to describe people who eat this way.

Lacto-ovo vegetarian
Vegetarians who include dairy and eggs in their diet are lacto-ovo vegetarians, sometimes abbreviated as LOV. Historically, most vegetarians in the United States have eaten this way, and much of what we know about vegan diets is actually extrapolated from studies of vegetarians.

Vegan
The word "vegan" was coined to describe a lifestyle that avoids all animal products for food, clothing, and personal care. It's based on ethical concerns regarding animals. However, a vegan diet—which includes no meat, fish, dairy, or eggs—is chosen by people for a variety of reasons, including issues regarding animal use as well as health and environmental considerations. Since this is a book about nutrition, when we use the word "vegan," we are referring to anyone who consumes a diet that includes only plant foods.

Our Journeys: How We Became Vegan Dietitians

Jack

I was nineteen years old and went on a fishing trip with my dad and grandfather. It consisted of putting out a number of lines at the same time, sitting back, and waiting for one to be tugged on. When a fish was reeled in, they put the fish in an empty watercooler, where it thrashed around for a good long time as it suffocated to death. I felt horrible about it and decided not to reel in any fish. I realized that if the fish were human, we would do all we could to save the person from such pain, but since it was a fish, no one cared. Yet the suffering seemed very similar. My grandfather and father were a bit confused by my reaction. Still, it took me another two years to stop eating fish!

Over the next two years, I read a few pages from *Animal Liberation*, which one of my philosophy professors showed me, which got me thinking, and then purchased *Animal Liberation*, which was a benefit album for People for the Ethical Treatment of Animals. I wrote to PETA for more information and started to learn about factory farms. The first food I gave up was eggs, followed by mammals and birds. My first couple of weeks not eating mammals and birds were hard because meat was very tempting, but soon I discovered some high-protein vegan foods and was satisfied with them. I gave up fish a few months later, and my only animal-product consumption at that point was one glass of cow's milk each day for calcium. When my chiropractor told me that I could get calcium from greens, I gave up dairy and went vegan in June of 1988.

After college, I became a full-time activist for animals, founded Vegan Outreach with Matt Ball, and spent two years traveling the country handing out our booklets on veganism to college students. In that time, I came across numerous people who said they had been vegan or vegetarian and had not been healthy. Due to this and all the other nutrition issues surrounding a vegan diet, I decided to become a registered dietitian so that I would know what I was talking about.

Ginny

When I headed off to college to become a dietitian, I was a carefree omnivore, chowing down happily on hamburgers and baked chicken. I've

continues

Our Journeys: How We Became Vegan Dietitians
continued

loved and felt great compassion for animals all my life, but for two and a half decades, it didn't occur to me that this had anything to do with how I should eat.

The little light bulb went on over my head just after I obtained my RD. I was newly married and cooking up all kinds of gourmet dinners, including—just for fun—some vegetarian ones. The first vegetarian cookbook I purchased was *Laurels' Kitchen*, and I credit it with nudging me onto the path toward ethical eating. Standing in the little kitchen in my apartment in Kalamazoo, Michigan, I opened it and read:

> This book is dedicated to a glossy black calf on his way to the slaughterhouse many years ago, whose eyes met those of someone who could understand their appeal and inspire us, and thousands of others like us, to give the gift of life.

Just like that, something clicked. Those simple words spoke volumes to me, and I knew right then and there that I wasn't going to eat animal flesh again.

Five years later, in 1989, I took a job working for the Physicians Committee for Responsible Medicine and once again made a huge leap in my understanding of what it means to eat ethically. As the staff dietitian, I did a lot of reading about dairy and egg production—and what I read absolutely stunned me. I learned that animals suffer just as much on dairy and egg farms as they do in meat production. I went "mostly vegan" and continued to refine my choices over the next several years, eventually removing all animal products from my diet as well as other parts of my life. I also dedicated my work to learning as much as possible about planning healthy animal-free diets. And my work as a writer and a consultant continues with that focus—sharing information about vegan nutrition and helping others make a safe and happy journey toward compassionate food choices.

Top Ten Myths about Vegan Diets

While vegan diets are gaining status more quickly than anyone could ever have imagined, they still sit well outside the mainstream. We have a big challenge in getting the message out that this way of eating is not only safe and healthful, but enjoyable and realistic too. At the same time, an enthusiasm for vegan eating among its proponents has given rise to unfortunate myths that cause some vegans to make poor food choices.

We're going to do some myth-busting in this book, and here are ten of the biggest ones that we'll tackle:

1. Vegans need less calcium than omnivores.
2. To reap the health benefits of a vegan diet, you need to avoid fat.
3. The healthiest vegan diets are based on 100 percent unprocessed whole foods.
4. People don't need to start taking vitamin B_{12} supplements until they have been vegan for three years.
5. If a vegan diet is good, then a raw-foods diet must be better.
6. Eating soy gives men female characteristics.
7. When you first go vegan, you'll experience unpleasant feelings from detoxing and withdrawal from animal products.
8. Vegan teens are at risk for developing eating disorders.
9. Plant proteins are missing some essential amino acids.
10. Vegans need to consume only 5 to 6 percent of their calories as protein.

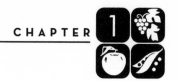

UNDERSTANDING VEGAN NUTRIENT NEEDS

Nutrition science was born in the early 1800s with the discovery of protein, carbohydrates, and fats. But long before that, humans knew a lot—strictly through trial and error—about food and health without actually understanding what the protective factors in foods were.

The first documented nutrition experiment was performed in 1747 by Dr. James Lind, a ship's doctor with the British Royal Navy. At the time, being a sailor was a dangerous occupation, not just because of storms and piracy, but because as many as half of all sailors who set out on long voyages died from scurvy. Theorizing that it had something to do with the lack of fruits and vegetables on board, Lind fed different diets to a small group of sailors and noted that those who consumed lemons and limes didn't get scurvy.

While the navy made good use of the information, ordering all British ships to carry limes, the reason that these foods were protective wasn't known for another two hundred years when researchers discovered vitamin C. (And while Lind got all the credit for discovering the cure for scurvy, Chinese sailors had been growing greens on their ships to ward off scurvy since at least the fifth century.)

As early as 1916, well before the discovery of many vitamins, nutritionists were recommending intake of certain "protective foods." The first RDAs were read over the radio to Americans in 1941 and have been updated and expanded a number of times since then.

Today, recommendations for individual nutrients are set by the Food and Nutrition Board (FNB) of the National Institute of Medicine. While these are official recommendations, the science behind them is sometimes still not entirely settled. In some cases, there isn't enough research for anything more than an educated guess. And actual individual requirements are affected by lifestyle, overall diet, and genetics, which means that it's impossible to pin down the exact nutrient requirements of any one person.

The recommendations are set at levels that are believed to meet the needs of the vast majority of Americans. Therefore, for any given nutrient, many Americans will need less than the recommended amount while others might need more. There can be exceptions, though. For example, many experts believe that current recommendations for vitamin D are far too low. And the debate about calcium recommendations is ongoing. We're also starting to hear questions from world experts about protein requirements; some think that they may fall short of actual needs.[1]

VEGANS AND THE RDAS

The dietary recommendations are aimed at omnivores and, in a few cases, nutrient needs might be higher for vegetarians and vegans. Protein requirements are believed to be slightly higher because plant protein isn't digested quite as well as protein from animals. It's a small difference and it's easily satisfied with vegan diets as long as calorie needs are met and your diet includes high-protein plant foods. Zinc needs may also be higher, and it's possible that some vegans have intakes that are less than optimal.

The situation for iron is a little more controversial. We'll see that vegans have higher requirements but how much higher is a subject of some debate. We've included the FNB recommendations for iron in the chart below, but we don't think that vegans should worry too much about getting this much iron. We'll talk much more about this issue in Chapter 6.

NUTRIENT INTAKE OF VEGANS: HOW DOES IT COMPARE TO RECOMMENDATIONS?

There isn't much available information about nutrient intakes of vegans, but a few studies show that vegans are likely to consume more of certain nutrients—vitamin C, thiamin, riboflavin, niacin, vitamin B_6, folate, and sometimes iron—than omnivores.[2] In contrast, many vegans have intakes of calcium and zinc that are lower than the recommendations. In the chart on pages 4 and 5, we've compared FNB recommendations to actual intakes of a group of British vegans.

GOOD DIETS ARE GOOD ADVOCACY

Whether you are already vegan or just starting to take steps in that direction, eliminating animal products from your lifestyle is an effective way to make a difference. It reduces animal suffering, removes your financial support for factory farming, and represents a stance against the use of animals. But in order to have the greatest impact possible, most of us who care about animals hope to influence others to go vegan as well.

Those who work for the meat, dairy, and egg industries would like to portray vegan diets as inadequate. So the last thing we want to do is give them any ammunition. Some vegans balk at the idea of taking vitamin B_{12} supplements, because they think it makes vegan diets appear inadequate. But taking a chance with nutrient deficiencies is the worst thing we can do for the image of vegan diets. For example, arguing that vegans have lower calcium needs than omnivores can cause some vegans to make poor choices for their bone health. Taking every precaution to make sure that we are healthy is one way to help others feel confident about going vegan.

Promoting veganism as a lifestyle that is practical, easy, and realistic is important, too. Time, convenience, and taste are primary factors in people's food choices. That's why overly restrictive diets can create the

NUTRIENT RECOMMENDATIONS FOR OMNIVORES AND VEGANS COMPARED TO INTAKES OF BRITISH VEGANS[3]

| | Recommended Intakes for Adults | | | | Intakes of British Vegans, 2003 | |
| | Omnivores | | Vegans | | | |
	MEN	WOMEN	MEN	WOMEN	MEN	WOMEN
Protein	0.36 grams per pound ideal body weight (or about 54 grams of protein per day for a person whose healthy body weight is 150 pounds.)	0.36 grams per pound ideal body weight	0.4 grams per pound ideal body weight (or around 60 grams of protein per day for a person whose healthy body weight is 150 pounds)	0.4 grams per pound ideal body weight	62 grams	56 grams
Vitamin A, RAE (retinol activity equivalents)	900	700				
Vitamin C, milligrams	90	70			155	169
Vitamin D, IUs	600	600				
Vitamin E, milligrams	15	15			16.1	14
Vitamin K, micrograms	120	90				
Thiamine, milligrams	1.2	1.1			2.3	2.1
Riboflavin, milligrams	1.3	1.1			2.3	2.1
Niacin, milligrams	16	14			23.9	21.1

continues

continued

| | Recommended Intakes for Adults | | | | Intakes of British Vegans, 2003 | |
| | Omnivores | | Vegans | | | |
	MEN	WOMEN	MEN	WOMEN	MEN	WOMEN
Vitamin B$_6$, milligrams	1.7	1.5			2.2	2.1
Folate, micrograms	400	400			431	412
Vitamin B$_{12}$, micrograms	2.4	2.4				
Calcium, milligrams	1000	1000			610	582
Copper, micrograms	900	900				
Chromium, micrograms	35	25				
Iodine, micrograms	150	150				
Iron, milligrams	8	18	14	33	15.3	14.1
Magnesium, milligrams	420	320			440	391
Selenium, micrograms	55	55				
Zinc, milligrams	11	8	16	12	7.9	7.2
Potassium, milligrams	4,700	4,700			3,937	3,817

wrong kind of image for veganism. Current trends among some vegans to give up more and more foods—added fats, cooked foods, and gluten—are counterproductive, especially because these dietary restrictions have few health benefits for most people. It's true that some people might have better success with weight control when they eat very little fat, but research suggests that diets containing small amounts of added fats or higher-fat foods can be even more beneficial for long-term weight control. And we'll look at why a little bit of unsaturated fat in the diet, especially monounsaturated fat, can be good for controlling and preventing chronic diseases.

Likewise, the idea behind a raw foods diet is based on a few scientific principles that are shaky at best. There is really no good evidence to suggest that eating all raw food is any better for you than eating a mix of raw and cooked whole plant foods. In fact, some of the beneficial compounds in foods, such as lycopene (an antioxidant in tomatoes that protects against prostate cancer), are available only when foods are cooked. The vitamin A precursor beta-carotene is more readily available from cooked foods as well and is also better absorbed in the presence of some fat. A raw foods diet can be helpful for weight control, since it has a lower caloric density, but this also means that it isn't appropriate for children.

A gluten-free diet is an absolute necessity for those who have celiac disease, a permanent intolerance to gluten. But this autoimmune disease affects only 1 percent of the population. That means that most vegans have no reason to eliminate gluten from their diets. In fact, some research suggests that gluten-free diets are associated with reductions in levels of beneficial gut bacteria and increased levels of harmful microbes. For those who don't have celiac disease, it may be beneficial to include some gluten in their diet. (Of course, those who have allergies, including non-celiac wheat allergy, need to adjust their diets accordingly.)

Promoting these additional restrictions that have *no known health advantage* for most people doesn't do anything to help animals or promote vegan diets. To the contrary, it creates an image of vegan diets that makes them look more difficult and less appealing. If we want others to follow our lead in adopting more compassionate food choices, it makes sense to avoid unnecessary restrictions and make vegan diets as accessible as possible.

The nutrition recommendations in this book, which are based on solid, current science, are aimed at making your vegan diet healthful and realistic. You'll see that it's easy to meet nutrient needs by eating a variety of cooked and raw plant foods, and it's also reasonable to plan some family meals using convenience products without compromising your health.

SUPPLEMENTS IN VEGAN DIETS

With the exception of vitamin B_{12}, it's possible to get all of the vitamins and minerals you need from plant foods. Depending on individual circumstances, though, vitamin supplements can provide an important way to meet nutrient needs, especially for vitamin D, iodine, calcium, and DHA.

While it's possible to purchase vitamin supplements that are food concentrates, many are synthetic—that is, they are synthesized in a laboratory. As long as they are well-digested, synthetic vitamins and minerals will do their job. In fact, in some cases they are a better source of nutrition than the food concentrates. For example, some "natural" vitamin B_{12} supplements are produced by companies that have not used proper testing standards and therefore, the B_{12} is not a reliable source of that nutrient.

The United States Pharmacopeia (USP) verifies the quality, purity, and potency of dietary supplements for companies that take part in their certification program. Supplements that display the "Dietary Supplement USP Verified" mark on labels have been tested to verify that they dissolve properly. (Vitamin and mineral supplements that don't carry the USP symbol may still be of high quality; it just means they haven't been certified.)

The supplements we recommend are for nutrients that can be low enough in vegan diets to lead to a deficiency. While a multivitamin can provide a number of these nutrients all at once, taking them as separate supplements will allow you to take only the supplements you need. A few things to keep in mind regarding supplements: First, most of us have sufficient stomach acid to dissolve supplements for thorough digestion. But if you have reason to believe that your stomach acid isn't strong, it's a good idea to crush or chew vitamin and mineral supplements. Also, supplements sometimes require a bit of attention to balance. For example, high doses of zinc can inhibit copper absorption. Taking 50 milligrams of zinc per day (the RDA is 8 to 11 milligrams) can cause a copper deficiency in just a few short weeks. This is one reason to rely on a well-balanced diet to provide enough nutrients and use supplements just to make up for any shortfall.

KEEPING NUTRITION SIMPLE

Humans require more than forty essential nutrients. Most people know that they need nutrients like vitamin C, protein, and calcium. But they may never have heard of the B vitamin biotin or the mineral vanadium and have no idea that they need to consume foods that provide these nutrients. And it's definitely not something you need to worry about. Most nutrients are so readily available in all different types of diets that we don't need to think about how to get them.

In this book, we're going to focus on just nine nutrients—protein, calcium, iron, zinc, iodine, alpha-linolenic acid, and vitamins B_{12}, A, and D. We'll briefly mention a handful of others and talk about DHA, an omega-3 fat that doesn't have essential nutrient status (meaning that, while a growing body of evidence suggests that it's important, it hasn't been established as a dietary essential). These are the nutrients that are of special interest to vegans and are the center of vegan nutrition. Getting enough of them isn't difficult. You just have to know how to do it.

Nutrient Recommendations: Some Terminology

Depending on the available research, determining precise needs is easier for some nutrients than for others. If researchers don't have enough data, or the findings are conflicting, it can be difficult to reach conclusions about optimal intakes. Therefore, current recommendations fall into several different categories, which are collectively known as the DRI (Dietary Reference Intakes):

Recommended Dietary Allowance (RDA): The amount of a nutrient that is believed to be sufficient to meet the needs of 97 to 98 percent of the population. It varies for different age groups and between men and women.

Adequate Intake (AI): When there isn't enough data to establish an RDA, the Institute of Medicine sets an AI, which is based on both studies and observations of what healthy populations consume. The recommendation for calcium, for example, is an AI because the data regarding calcium needs is conflicting.

Tolerable Upper Intake Level (UL): This is the maximum daily intake of a nutrient that is likely to be safe. Some nutrients can be extremely toxic at higher than normal levels, although excessive intakes are almost always associated with supplements.

Daily Values (DV): These are values used strictly for food labeling purposes and they are based on much older RDAs. The amounts of vitamins and minerals in a food are listed as a percent of the DV. For example, the DV for calcium is 1000 milligrams, so if a food contains 10 percent of the DV for calcium per serving, it provides 100 milligrams of calcium. The problem is that without knowing what the DV is for a specific nutrient—and the food label doesn't tell you—it's hard to know exactly what these numbers mean. As we discuss the nutrients that are especially relevant to vegans in the next several chapters, we'll give you the information you need to decipher food labels.

UNDERSTANDING NUTRITION RESEARCH

The amount of nutrition information in the media and on the Internet is staggering. Much of it is conflicting and often studies looking at the same question come up with completely different answers.

In fact, for essentially all heavily researched areas, you can build a case for just about anything by picking and choosing the studies that support your point. Some advocates do this to make vegan diets look more beneficial. And some vegan detractors pick a completely different set of studies to make vegan diets look bad.

The key to understanding nutrition research is to look at the *entire body of evidence* and see what *most studies* say. Rarely can a single study provide a definitive answer to a question. There are always inconsistencies and there are always study flaws. In addition, different types of studies carry different weight. So the strengths and weaknesses of certain types of studies have to be balanced against the strengths and weaknesses of others.

TYPES OF STUDIES

Weakest Evidence

These types of studies don't provide conclusive evidence but are conducted primarily to determine if further research is warranted.

- Neither *in vitro* (studies conducted in test tubes or cell culture often using single cells) nor *animal studies* can serve as the basis for conclusions about diet and disease. Aside from any ethical considerations and despite their widespread use, findings about nutrition from animal studies often can't predict what is going to happen in humans.
- A *case study* is an observation about one or perhaps several patient histories and their treatment and disease outcomes that is published in a scientific journal. Often these types of reports can

be used as a basis for hypothesis generation, but they don't provide definitive answers. In contrast, if a report isn't published in a peer-reviewed journal, it is merely an anecdote and has little or no value in contributing to nutrition knowledge. A great deal of nutrition information on the Internet and in books—including books by doctors and other health professionals—is based on anecdotes rather than actual science.

- *Ecological* (also called correlational) studies compare food habits and disease rates among different groups of people. One ecological study that is familiar to many vegans looked at rates of hip fracture and protein consumption in different countries.[4] The results showed that as protein intake increases, so does the rate of hip fracture. But contrary to popular opinion, that study didn't show that high protein intake causes weak bones. (We talk more about why that is in Chapter 4.) It did set the stage for clinical studies on how protein might impact calcium metabolism.

  Another type of ecological study is the migration study, which looks at what happens to the health of people when they relocate and acquire the food and lifestyle habits of their adopted homeland. These kinds of studies can help show whether risk for certain diseases is related more to genetics or lifestyle.

  Ecological studies are riddled with problems because there are many factors that affect health outcomes and these can't be completely controlled for in the analysis of the data. Additionally, individual food intakes can only be roughly estimated.

Better Evidence: Epidemiologic Research

Epidemiologic studies can establish that two factors occur together but not that one causes the other. They are prone to *confounding variables*, which means that there might be unidentified issues that cause two factors to be associated. For example, if researchers find out that people with low fruit intakes are more likely to get cancer, it seems logical that fruit is protective against this disease. But what if those who don't eat fruit also don't exercise? It's difficult to establish whether it is lack of fruit or lack of exercise or a combination of both that raises the risk.

Ecological studies, discussed above, are the weakest type of epidemiological studies. The following three types of epidemiology provide stronger evidence.

- *Retrospective studies* compare past eating habits between people with and without a particular disease. For example, if people with heart disease are more likely to have eaten a diet high in saturated fat, we might conclude that saturated fat has something to do with heart disease. The main drawback of these studies for nutrition research is that people's memories of their previous diet can be faulty, especially if it has changed over the years.
- *Cross-sectional* studies compare eating habits and disease rates in groups of people at one moment in time. One problem is that people who have recently become ill may have recently changed their diet.
- *Prospective* (also called cohort) studies follow large numbers of people who are (usually) healthy when the study begins. As the population is followed, eating patterns of those who eventually get a disease are compared to those who do not. These studies require a lot of subjects—numbering in the tens of thousands—and take place over a long period of time, but they carry the most weight among epidemiologists

Best Evidence: Clinical Trials

The *randomized controlled trial* (RCT) is the gold standard in nutrition research. It's the most credible type of study because it randomly assigns people to different groups and then controls what they eat. Ideally, the study is double-blinded; that is, the subjects don't know whether they are in the test group or the control group. And when the researchers collect the data, they don't know which group it came from until all the data has been collected and analyzed. The effects of different supplements or foods on disease markers, like cholesterol or bone density, can be studied this way. These studies can be very powerful, and ideally, everything we want to know about nutrition would be tested through RCTs. Unfortunately, they are expensive and complex, which is why they are often smaller in size and shorter in duration than is ideal.

OTHER CONSIDERATIONS

A Word about Statistics

Statistical analyses are always performed to eliminate the probability that different outcomes occurred by random chance. Generally, a finding is *statistically significant* if there is less than a 5 percent chance that it occurred by chance. When studies are small in size, it becomes difficult to show statistical significance. Even if there appears to be an effect of a treatment or differences between groups, if the differences and treatment are not statistically significant, scientists conclude that there was no effect.

One way to make good use of the data from smaller studies is to do a *meta-analysis*. This is a statistical analysis of a large number of studies for the purpose of integrating the findings. It is often done to compensate for the small size of individual studies.

Peer Review

Scientific journals make sure that studies are credible and worth publishing by having them reviewed by other researchers qualified to do so. The reviewers can recommend that the study be published or not, based on what they think of the study design and other factors.

Who Paid for the Study?

Most nutrition research is funded by the government, but some is paid for by industry. It probably doesn't matter as much as you might think.

The results are what they are and the sponsoring party can't change them. The only real advantage is that they get a peek at the data before it is published; that way their PR department can be ready to issue a press release.

In conclusion, we can make educated statements about vegan nutrition only by looking at what most of the studies say (rather than drawing conclusions from individual studies) and by focusing on the studies that are likely to yield the most reliable information. It's also important that studies are published in peer-reviewed journals.

CHAPTER 2

PROTEIN FROM PLANTS

Nutrition researchers declared more than thirty years ago that plant foods can provide adequate protein.[1] But "where do you get your protein?" is a question that most vegans have heard more times than they can count. Many of the questions about protein in plant-based diets stem from confusion over what it means for proteins to be "complete."

COMPLETE AND INCOMPLETE PROTEINS

Proteins are made of chains of twenty different amino acids. Some amino acids can be made by the body (generally from other amino acids) and therefore we don't need a dietary source of them. Others—the *essential amino acids* (EAAs)—must be supplied by the diet.

Proteins in the human body tend to have a consistent ratio of EAAs. Because the percentage of EAAs in animal products and soybeans are a close match to those in the human body, proteins from these foods are considered "complete." Plant foods like grains, beans and nuts have a lower percentage of at least one essential amino acid, making them "incomplete." For example, beans (other than soybeans) are low in the EAA methionine, and grains are low in lysine. But when grains and beans are consumed together, their amino acid profiles complement each other and produce a mix that is "complete" and therefore a good match to the body's needs.

In the early 1970s, the idea that vegetarian meals should contain these specific complementary pairings was popularized in *Diet for a Small Planet* by Frances Moore Lappé.[2] Today we know that the theory about what happens when protein foods are combined in this way wasn't wrong; it just turned out to be unnecessary. Newer research has shown that the body maintains its own storage supply of the essential amino acids.[3] We need to keep replenishing that storage with all of the amino acids, and so it's important to eat a variety of plant foods. But the old idea that certain combinations of plant foods—the complementary pairings—must be consumed together isn't true.

While fruit is extremely low in protein, and oils don't provide any, all other plant foods contain protein. One common misconception is that plant foods are completely without one or more amino acids. That's not true. All plant sources of protein contain at least some of every essential amino acid. In fact, you could get enough protein and all of the essential amino acids by eating just one type of food like pinto beans. You'd need to eat a lot of them, though—about four cups per day. That's not practical, partly because it would be boring, but also because all those beans are likely to displace foods that are needed to satisfy other nutrient requirements. So eating a variety of protein sources makes better nutritional sense.

PROTEIN RDA FOR VEGANS

Protein needs are calculated on the basis of healthy (or "ideal") body weight—that is, what a person with a healthy amount of body fat weighs. Scientists use the metric system, so U.S. protein needs are determined using your healthy weight in kilograms.

The protein RDA for adults is 0.8 grams of protein per kilogram of ideal body weight, but along with most other vegan dietitians, we recommend a slightly higher protein intake for vegans. This is because plant proteins are not digested as well as animal proteins.[4] Since both cooking and processing often improve protein digestibility, this may be less of an issue for vegans who consume more foods like tofu or veggie meats made from processed soy protein. For those who are depending on whole foods like legumes, nuts, and grains for most of their protein, the digestibility factor comes into play.

It's not a big difference, but vegans should strive for a protein intake of 0.9 grams per kilogram of body weight. For ease of calculation, this translates to around 0.4 grams of protein per pound of healthy body weight. So a vegan whose healthy weight is 150 pounds would need 60 grams of protein (150 x 0.4) per day.

Since protein needs vary considerably among individuals, the RDA is designed to cover the needs of 97 percent of the population and is therefore more than what many people need. Without any way of knowing where you fall on the protein-need spectrum, and because recent research suggests that protein recommendations could be too low,[5] it's a good idea to play it safe and aim for the RDA.

For children and teens, we would use an RDA aimed at the needs of different age groups and calculated specifically for vegans.

PROTEIN RECOMMENDATIONS FOR YOUNG VEGANS

Age (years)	Females (grams/day)	Males (grams/day)
1–2	18–19	18–19
2–3	18–21	18–21
4–6	26–28	26–28
7–10	31–34	31–34
11–14	51–55	50–54
15–18	50–55	66–73

MEETING PROTEIN NEEDS ON A VEGAN DIET:
THE IMPORTANCE OF LEGUMES

While the chart on page 19 shows that many plant foods are good protein sources, legumes are especially rich in protein. Legumes include beans, peas, lentils, soyfoods (like tofu, soymilk, and veggie meats), and peanuts. (Most people think of peanuts as nuts, but they are botanically legumes and, from a nutritional standpoint, they have more in common with pinto beans and lentils than walnuts and pecans.) Our food guide specifies at least three to four servings per day of these foods. A serving is pretty modest: ½ cup of cooked beans, ½ cup of tofu or tempeh, a one-ounce veggie burger, one cup of soymilk, or two tablespoons of peanut butter. Planning menus that include these foods isn't difficult, and we give you several tips for doing so in Chapter 7.

In addition to being protein-rich, these foods are the only good plant sources—with a few exceptions—of the essential amino acid lysine. A diet that gets most of its protein from grains, nuts, and vegetables is likely to be too low in lysine. And while some popular resources suggest that very low protein intakes—as little as 5 to 6 percent of total calories—can meet our nutritional needs, it's actually difficult to get enough lysine (or total protein) on a diet that isn't more protein-dense.

You can get a rough idea of how much lysine you need by multiplying your weight (in pounds) by 19. This calculation includes a small factor that makes up for the slightly lower digestibility of protein from whole plant foods. For example, a person weighing 140 pounds would need 2,660 milligrams of lysine per day. The chart on page 21 shows that the best sources of lysine are legumes, quinoa, pistachios, and cashews.

If you follow our recommendations to consume at least three to four servings of legumes per day, you'll meet lysine needs with ease. That doesn't mean that beans, peanuts, and soyfoods are absolutely essential in vegan diets. While it is difficult to meet protein and lysine needs without them, it's possible, and we provide guidance on how in Chapter 7, when we look at meal planning guidelines for vegans.

PROTEIN CONTENT OF SELECTED VEGAN FOODS

Food	Protein content (in grams)
Legumes and soyfoods (½ cup cooked unless otherwise noted)	
Black beans	7.6
Garbanzo beans	7.5
Kidney beans	8.1
Lentils	8.9
Navy beans	7.5
Pinto beans	7.7
Seitan*, 3 ounces	22.5
Soybeans	14.3
Soy-free protein powder, Naturade brand, ⅓ cup	22
Soy protein powder, Naturade brand, ⅓ cup (contains protein from peas, potatoes, and spirulina with extra amounts of the essential amino acids lysine and methionine)	23
Tempeh	15.5
Textured vegetable protein	11
Tofu, firm	10–20**
Tofu, soft	8–10
Vegetarian baked beans	6
Veggie meats, 1 ounce	6–18
Vegetable milks (1 cup)	
Almond milk	1
Hempseed milk	2
Rice milk	1
Soymilk	5–10
Nuts and seeds	
Almonds, ¼ cup	7.3
Almond butter, 2 tablespoons	7
Brazil nuts, ¼ cup	4.7
Cashews, ¼ cup	5.2
Flaxseed, 1 teaspoon ground	0.5
Peanuts, ¼ cup	8.6

*Seitan is wheat protein. It is not a legume, but because of its high protein content, it is usually grouped with legumes and soyfoods for meal-planning purposes.

**Firm tofu is usually higher in protein than soft tofu, but the protein content of different brands and types of tofu varies widely.

continues

continued

PROTEIN CONTENT OF SELECTED VEGAN FOODS

Food	Protein content (in grams)
Nuts and seeds (continued)	
Peanut butter, 2 tablespoons	8
Pecans, ¼ cup	2.5
Pine nuts, 2 tablespoons	2.4
Pistachios, ¼ cup	6.4
Pumpkin seeds, 2 tablespoons	4.4
Sesame seeds, 2 tablespoons	2.7
Sunflower seeds, 2 tablespoons	3.1
Tahini, 2 tablespoons	5
Walnuts, ¼ cup	4.4
Grains (½ cup cooked unless otherwise noted)	
Barley	1.7
Millet	3
Oatmeal	3
Pasta	4
Quinoa	4.0
Rice, brown	2.5
Rice, white	2.0
Taco shell, 1 medium	1.0
Whole wheat bread	2–6
Vegetables (½ cup cooked or 1 cup raw)	
Broccoli	2.3
Carrots	0.6
Cauliflower	1.1
Collards	2
Corn	2.3
Eggplant	0.4
Green beans	1.2
Kale	1.3
Mushrooms	1.7
Potato, 1 baked	4.5
Spinach	2.6 (3.8 for frozen)
Sweet potato	2.2
Turnips	0.5
Turnip greens	0.8

LYSINE CONTENT OF SELECTED PLANT FOODS

Food	Amount of Lysine (in milligrams)
Protein powders	
Naturade soy-free protein powder, ⅓ cup	1,455
Naturade soy protein powder, ⅓ cup	1,552
Soyfoods	
Edamame, ½ cup	577.5
Soymilk, 1 cup	439
Tofu, firm, ½ cup	582
Legumes	
Black beans, ½ cup	523
Garbanzo beans (chickpeas), ½ cup	486.5
Kidney beans, ½ cup	526.5
Lentils, ½ cup	623.5
Peanut butter, 2 tablespoons	290
Peanuts, ¼ cup	310
Refried pinto beans, ½ cup	475
Nuts and seeds	
Almonds, ¼ cup	205
Cashews, ¼ cup	280
Pecans, ¼ cup	78
Pistachios, ¼ cup	367
Walnuts, ¼ cup	124
Grains	
Bread, white, 1 slice	56
Bread, whole wheat, 1 slice	85
Oatmeal, ½ cup cooked	158
Potato (white), ½ medium	131.5
Quinoa, ½ cup	221
Rice, brown, ½ cup	86
Rice, white, ½ cup	80
Spaghetti, white, ½ cup	63.5
Spaghetti, whole wheat, ½ cup	82.5
Tortilla, flour, 1 medium	98
Vegetables	
Broccoli, ½ cup	117
Corn, ½ cup	116
Romaine lettuce, 1 cup raw shredded	58
Spinach, ½ cup cooked	164
Fruits	
Banana, 1 medium	59
Orange, 1 medium	62
Strawberries, whole, 1 cup	37

VEGAN PROTEIN: MEALS THAT DELIVER

It's easy to build meals that pack a substantial protein punch. Each of these meals provides at least 20 grams of protein.

EASY OATMEAL BREAKFAST

- ▸ 1 cup of oatmeal with ½ cup soymilk
- ▸ 1 slice whole-wheat bread with 2 tablespoons almond butter

■ Total protein: 20.5 grams

INDONESIAN TEMPEH WITH PEANUT SAUCE

- ▸ 1 cup of rice
- ▸ ½ cup tempeh
- ▸ ¼ cup sesame tahini sauce
- ▸ 1½ cups steamed broccoli

■ Total protein: 35 grams

BEAN AND BEEF TACO DINNER

- ▸ 2 taco shells
- ▸ ½ cup refried beans
- ▸ ¼ cup veggie "ground beef" cooked in tomato sauce
- ▸ Chopped tomatoes and lettuce
- ▸ 1 cup steamed spinach

■ Total protein: 20 grams

PASTA PRIMAVERA

- ▸ 1 cup pasta
- ▸ ½ cup garbanzo beans
- ▸ 2 tablespoons pine nuts
- ▸ 1 cup chopped broccoli
- ▸ ½ cup roasted red pepper strips

■ Total protein: 23 grams

LUNCH ON THE GO

- ▸ Instant lentil soup with 2 tablespoons pumpkin seeds
- ▸ 1 slice whole-wheat bread with mashed avocado

■ Total protein: 21 grams

INADEQUATE INTAKES

Overt protein deficiency is rare among Americans and occurs in other parts of the world where people don't have enough food. Many vegan advocates point out that people don't end up in hospitals because of a protein deficiency. It's true that in countries where food is abundant, acute deficiency of protein doesn't occur. But diets that are marginal in protein—not quite deficient, but not quite optimal—can result in loss of muscle mass, poor bone health, and compromised immunity. And those kinds of problems do occur in the United States.

We'd like to say that vegans never need to worry about protein, but that isn't entirely true. There are a few situations where vegans may fall short on meeting their protein needs.

Vegan diets that are low in protein-rich foods like legumes are likely to be too low in protein. And because low-calorie diets raise protein requirements, people who are dieting or simply not eating enough for other reasons (like chronic illness) may need to boost their intake of protein-rich foods like legumes or soyfoods.

Obviously, junk-food vegan diets—those based on potato chips, French fries, and soft drinks—can be too low in protein (and too low in just about everything else that you need to be healthy).

And extreme versions of vegan diets, such as raw foods or fruitarian regimens, are often low (or completely lacking) in the higher-protein plant foods like legumes and soyfoods and can lead to a marginal protein intake. That's one reason these types of diets are not recommended for children.

DO VEGANS GET ADEQUATE TRYPTOPHAN?

One common belief, often voiced by critics of vegan diets, is that plant foods don't provide adequate tryptophan. This essential amino acid is needed to make the neurotransmitter serotonin, and low levels of serotonin are linked to depression. Meat is higher in tryptophan than plants, but a well-balanced vegan diet is almost guaranteed to provide more than enough of this amino acid. The FNB recommends 5 milligrams of tryptophan for every kilogram of healthy body weight. Adding in a factor for plant protein digestion, this translates to a vegan RDA of 5.5 milligrams per kilogram of body weight or 2.5 milligrams of tryptophan per pound.

For example, a vegan who weighs 130 pounds would need 325 milligrams of tryptophan, which is easily provided on a vegan diet. A diet that includes one cup of black beans, ½ cup of tofu and one cup of brown rice would provide nearly 400 milligrams of tryptophan.

In fact, eating foods that are very high in protein, like meat, doesn't necessarily increase the amount of tryptophan in the brain. That's because high levels of other amino acids in these foods block absorption of tryptophan from the blood into the brain. Eating foods like legumes that provide both protein and carbohydrates can actually enhance the passage of tryptophan into the brain.[6]

TRYPTOPHAN CONTENT OF SELECTED VEGAN FOODS

Food	Tryptophan (in millligrams)
Tofu, ½ cup	155
Oatmeal, ½ cup	118
Soymilk, 1 cup	105
Black beans, ½ cup cooked	90
Peanut butter, 2 tablespoons	78
Garbanzo beans, ½ cup cooked	70
Quinoa, ½ cup cooked	48
Brown rice, ½ cup cooked	29
Broccoli, ½ cup cooked	24

TIPS FOR MEETING VEGAN PROTEIN NEEDS

- Consume adequate calories to maintain a healthful weight. If your calorie intake is low because you are dieting or for any other reason, you may need to add a few additional protein-rich foods to your menus.
- Eat a variety of plant foods every day.
- Follow the guidelines in The Vegan Food Guide in Chapter 7 and aim for at least three to four servings of legumes in your daily menu. A serving is ½ cup cooked beans, ½ cup tofu or tempeh, ¼ cup peanuts, one cup soymilk, or 2 tablespoons peanut butter.
- If beans give you discomfort from gas production, choose more lentils and split peas (they're less gassy) and include some veggie meats, tofu, or tempeh in your menus.
- If you include plant milks in your diet, choose soymilk at least some of the time. Milks made from almonds, hempseed, and rice are low in protein.

CHAPTER 3

VITAMIN B$_{12}$:
The Gorilla in the Room

You may have heard that vitamin B$_{12}$ is a controversial topic among vegans. But among nutrition professionals (including those of us who specialize in vegan diets), there is no controversy at all: All vegans need to take a vitamin B$_{12}$ supplement or consume foods that are fortified with this nutrient.

Vitamin B$_{12}$ is needed for cell division and formation of healthy red blood cells. It's also needed to produce myelin, the protective sheath around nerve fibers. Overt B$_{12}$ deficiency can produce a condition called macrocytic or megaloblastic anemia, in which blood cells don't divide and reproduce normally. Deficiency can also result in nerve damage. But because B$_{12}$ is also involved in metabolism of fat and protein, a marginal intake may increase the risk for certain chronic conditions like heart disease.

The scientific name for vitamin B$_{12}$ is cobalamin because the B$_{12}$ molecule contains the mineral cobalt at the center of its structure. Commercial preparations of vitamin B$_{12}$ used in supplements and fortified foods are called cyanocobalamin. This supplemental form is converted in the body to vitamin B$_{12}$ coenzymes, which are the compounds needed for B$_{12}$ activity. Some people prefer to take supplements of vitamin B$_{12}$ that are already in the form of the coenzyme methylcobalamin, which doesn't require any conversion for some of its uses. But because there are questions about the stability of methylcobalamin, supplements must contain much higher amounts and there is less available research on their effects on B_{12} status. The recommendations we make in this chapter are based on supplements and fortified foods that utilize cyanocobalamin.

VEGAN SOURCES OF VITAMIN B_{12}

All of the vitamin B_{12} in the world is made by bacteria, and that includes bacteria living in the digestive tracts of animals and humans. It seems like we could just use what these bacteria produce, but they are too far down in the intestines to be of any use to us. We absorb vitamin B_{12} in our small intestine; the bacteria producing it live in our large intestine.

There are also molecules that are very similar to vitamin B_{12} but that have no true vitamin activity for humans. These are inactive B_{12} analogues. Most methods for measuring vitamin B_{12} in foods don't differentiate between true vitamin B_{12} and the inactive analogues. That's been a source of confusion for a long time. Foods like fermented soy products, tofu, sourdough bread, and some sea vegetables have all been credited at one time or another as good sources of vitamin B_{12}. But studies show that what they really contain are primarily inactive analogues.[1] There is a double risk associated with depending on these foods for vitamin B_{12}, because the inactive analogues can actually block the activity of true vitamin B_{12}.[2]

Some companies may claim that a food contains active vitamin B_{12} even though the testing methods they use can't discern between active B_{12} and inactive analogues. Currently, the only way to know if a food contains active vitamin B_{12} is to feed it to humans and look for vitamin B_{12} activity. The standard way to do this is to see how different foods affect levels of a compound called methylmalonic acid (MMA). MMA levels increase in B_{12} deficiency, and consuming foods that contain active vitamin B_{12} causes those levels to drop. Many foods that are commonly believed to be good sources of vitamin B_{12} actually have no effect on MMA levels, which means that they contain primarily inactive analogues.

Plants have no need for B$_{12}$, which is why they usually don't contain any. Occasionally, a plant food might be "contaminated" with an inactive B$_{12}$ analogue. That is, it contains vitamin B$_{12}$ by accident. For example, the "starter" used to make tempeh, which is a fermented soyfood, might accidentally contain B$_{12}$-producing bacteria. Seaweed might pick up bacteria that produce B$_{12}$-analogues. There is some evidence that sea vegetables such as chlorella, dulse, and nori contain vitamin B$_{12}$, but again, these haven't been shown to be reliable and significant sources of the active vitamin.[3]

Most humans get vitamin B$_{12}$ by eating animal products. Animals such as cows and other true herbivores are able to absorb the vitamin B$_{12}$ produced in their intestines by bacteria. Others, including many primate species, eat at least small amounts of animal products (including insects) or feces, which can be a good source of B$_{12}$.

It would follow that soil and water that are contaminated with human or animal waste should contain vitamin B$_{12}$, and they might. But while there is speculation about this among research scientists, there is no direct evidence for it. One paper that has gained support among some vegan groups was actually just an abstract in *Science* magazine from 1950 by researchers with the New York Botanical Gardens. The methods used didn't determine whether the B$_{12}$ was active. A more recent finding that plants could take up vitamin B$_{12}$ from manure-treated soil didn't show whether the B$_{12}$ was active vitamin or inactive analogue. And it doesn't really matter because the amounts were so tiny that they didn't have any nutritional significance.[4]

Humans definitely evolved to get by on pretty low intakes of vitamin B$_{12}$. We have a rather complex physiological way of recycling it, and we also can store relatively large amounts in our livers—sometimes enough to prevent overt deficiency for as long as three years. As a result, some vegan advocates insist that no one needs to worry about vitamin B$_{12}$ until they have been a vegan for several years and that we can get by with taking supplements just "once in a while." We think this approach is a mistake for a couple of reasons.

First, not everyone has a three-year B_{12} supply. It depends on what your diet has been like over time. Building up generous B_{12} stores can take many years of consuming the vitamin in quantities that exceed daily needs. If you have been eating a mostly plant-based or lacto-ovo vegetarian diet before becoming vegan—that is, a diet that is more moderate in animal foods than what most Americans eat—your vitamin B_{12} stores may be relatively low. Some people may find themselves running through their B_{12} supply in just a few months. In addition, vitamin B_{12} stores may not be sufficient to prevent mild, marginal-type deficiencies, as we'll see below.

VITAMIN B_{12} DEFICIENCY

Overt deficiency occurs when vitamin B_{12} stores drop to near zero. The megaloblastic anemia that occurs with B_{12} deficiency is reversible with vitamin B_{12} therapy. Sometimes B_{12} deficiency anemia is "masked" by the vitamin folic acid (also called folate), which can step in and do vitamin B_{12}'s job. So you can be deficient in vitamin B_{12} but not have anemia if your diet is high in folate.

This may sound like a good thing, but it's not since folic acid won't prevent the nerve damage that can occur with B_{12} deficiency. If B_{12} intake is low and folate intake is high, B_{12} deficiency can go unnoticed until it progresses to a more advanced stage. It's an important issue for vegans since they typically have a high intake of folate, which is found in leafy greens, oranges, and beans.[5]

The neurological damage that can result from a B_{12} deficiency typically begins with tingling in the hands and feet and can progress to far more serious symptoms. Often the symptoms can be reversed, but some neurological damage can be permanent. This is especially true in babies born to mothers who don't have adequate vitamin B_{12} intake during pregnancy.

The anemia and neurological symptoms associated with overt B_{12} deficiency are fairly obvious. But a second type of "mild" deficiency doesn't have acute symptoms. It does its damage over time—often decades—and is only detected through medical tests. When B$_{12}$ levels in the blood start to drop, levels of an amino acid called homocysteine begin to rise. Homocysteine may damage blood vessels and nervous tissue and many studies have linked high levels to an increased risk for heart disease, stroke, and early death.[6] Elevated homocysteine may also be related to Alzheimer's disease[7] and neural tube defects in the developing embryo.[8]

Research shows that vegetarians and vegans who supplement with vitamin B$_{12}$ have healthy levels of homocysteine. Those who don't take supplements have high homocysteine levels.[9] These findings present strong evidence that vegans who don't use supplements—and who insist that they feel fine—may be damaging their health over the long term. (Folate and vitamin B$_6$ also affect the vitamin homocysteine, but most vegans get plenty of those.)

While this might sound like vitamin B$_{12}$ is a big problem for vegans, it's an issue that's so easily resolved it shouldn't be a concern. In fact, it's a concern only when vegans don't get good advice about vitamin B$_{12}$ or don't want to use supplements or fortified foods.

We think that vegans actually have the advantage when it comes to vitamin B$_{12}$. Here is why: As people age, no matter what type of diet they follow, their ability to absorb vitamin B$_{12}$ found naturally in foods begins to decline.[10] Vitamin B$_{12}$ in animal foods is bound to protein, and the decrease in stomach acid that tends to occur in older people makes it harder to release B$_{12}$ from the protein so it can be absorbed. Because the vitamin B$_{12}$ in supplements and fortified foods is not bound to protein, it is more easily absorbed by older people. For this reason, the FNB recommends that all people over age fifty get at least half of the RDA for B$_{12}$ from some combination of supplements and fortified foods. Many older people may not know this, but vegans who are paying attention to good nutrition advice are already using vitamin B$_{12}$ supplements or fortified foods.

SUPPLEMENTING VERSUS MONITORING

It has been suggested that anyone who is worried about whether or not they should take supplements should simply get their B$_{12}$ levels tested. But that doesn't make any sense. You don't want to wait until your levels are low to start supplementing. And if your levels are normal, you should supplement in order to maintain them. There is no reason not to take supplements. They are inexpensive and safe. So you can have your B_{12} levels tested if you want, but regardless of the results, you should follow the advice about vitamin B_{12} supplements and fortified foods we've outlined below.

MEETING VITAMIN B_{12} NEEDS

There are a couple of important things to keep in mind about supplementing with B_{12}. First, B_{12} supplements should be either chewable or sublingual (dissolving under the tongue) since research shows that, in some people, B_{12} isn't well absorbed from pills that are swallowed whole.

Also, the body is used to getting little bits of vitamin B_{12} here and there throughout the day. When confronted with a big dose of B_{12}, it absorbs just a tiny fraction of the whole amount. So when you take vitamin B_{12} infrequently, you need rather large amounts in order to get enough. The RDA for vitamin B_{12} is just 2.4 micrograms for adults. But if you are getting your daily dose from a supplement, you may need as much as 25 to 100 micrograms. And if you supplement just two or three times a week, you may need 1,000 micrograms each time.

If you have not had a regular source of vitamin B_{12} for some time, we recommend taking 2,000 micrograms every day for two weeks before beginning the regular supplementation schedule as follows.

To meet your vitamin B_{12} requirements on a vegan diet do any *one* of the following:

- Consume two servings per day of fortified foods providing 1.5 to 2.5 micrograms of vitamin B_{12} each.
- Take a daily vitamin B_{12} supplement of at least 25 micrograms (25 to 100 micrograms is a good range).
- Take a supplement of 1,000 micrograms of vitamin B_{12} three times a week.

GETTING B$_{12}$ FROM FORTIFIED FOODS

Plant foods are reliable sources of active vitamin B$_{12}$ only if they are fortified with the vitamin. On food labels, the Daily Value for vitamin B$_{12}$ is 6 micrograms. So if a food provides 25 percent of the Daily Value, it contains 1.5 micrograms.

Nutritional yeast is a popular choice with many vegans. Its cheesy-yeasty flavor is great mixed into bean and grain dishes or sprinkled over popcorn. Nutritional yeast is grown on a nutrient-rich culture and contains only the nutrients that are in that culture. So don't assume that every type of nutritional yeast is a good source of vitamin B$_{12}$. Red Star brand Vegetarian Support Formula is a good vitamin B$_{12}$–rich choice that is widely available, often in the bulk food section of natural foods markets. Brewer's yeast is a by-product of beer making and is not a good source of vitamin B$_{12}$. Neither is the active yeast used in bread making.

VITAMIN B$_{12}$ CONTENT OF FORTIFIED VEGAN FOODS

Food	Vitamin B$_{12}$ Content (µg)
Nutritional yeast, Vegetarian Support Formula, 1 tablespoon	4.0
Veggie "meat" analogues, fortified	1.0–3.0 (varies by brand)
Soymilk, fortified, 1 cup	1.2–2.9 (varies by brand)
Protein bar, fortified	1.0–2.0 (varies by brand)
Marmite yeast extract, 1 teaspoon	0.9

VITAMIN B$_{12}$ FACTS

- The vitamin B$_{12}$ in supplements comes from bacterial cultures—never from animal products.

- B_{12} pills should be chewed or allowed to dissolve under the tongue.
- Seaweed (e.g., algae, nori, spirulina), brewer's yeast, tempeh, or "living" vitamin supplements that use plants as a source of B_{12} don't contain any vitamin B_{12} or have only inactive analogues.
- Neither rainwater nor organically grown, unwashed vegetables are a reliable source of vitamin B_{12}.
- If you rely on fortified food sources of vitamin B_{12}, it is best to have at least two fortified food sources on hand in case a particular batch of a food contains vitamin B_{12} that is somehow damaged. Do not rely solely on one type of fortified food.
- About 2 percent of older people can't absorb B_{12}. This disease is called *pernicious anemia*. Being vegan has nothing to do with this condition, but if you are supplementing regularly with vitamin B_{12} and still suspect that you have symptoms of vitamin B_{12} deficiency, such as extreme fatigue or neurological problems, then by all means get your B_{12} levels tested. Pernicious anemia is treated with vitamin B_{12} injections.

IS A VEGAN DIET NATURAL?

It wouldn't be right to ignore the four-hundred-pound gorilla in the room, so let's ask the obvious question: Since vitamin B_{12} is not found in plant foods and vegans must take supplements, doesn't that make a vegan diet unnatural?

Many vegans have bent over backwards to convince themselves and others that humans evolved as vegans and that supplemental vitamin B_{12} is only needed because we have moved so far away from our natural environment. But there is a tremendous amount of evidence that humans evolved eating some animal products. While B_{12} is not needed in large amounts, it may take more than can be picked up from unwashed produce to sustain optimal levels. That's especially true during pregnancy and lactation, when a woman needs to consume enough B_{12} for her own needs and to pass on to her baby.

In fact, adding small amounts of animal products to the diet has been shown not to cure B$_{12}$ deficiency. At least one study showed that some lacto-ovo vegetarians may have vitamin B$_{12}$ status that is similar to that of vegans when neither group supplemented.[11] If consuming small amounts of animal foods doesn't improve vitamin B$_{12}$ status, then it is unlikely that inadvertently ingesting B$_{12}$ from unwashed produce would be enough to sustain vegans through the life cycle in a pre-vitamin-supplement culture.

Paleontology student Robert Mason, who writes the PaleoVeganology website, says this about the evolution of human diets: "This touches on the issue of how vegans should handle the caveman argument. Many of us are tempted to strain credulity and torture the evidence to 'prove' humans are 'naturally' vegan. This is a trap, and one into which carnists (especially paleo-dieters) would love us to fall; the evidence isn't on our side. There's no doubt that hominids ate meat. . . . The argument for veganism has always been primarily ethical, and ought to remain that way. It's based on a concern for the future, not an obsession about the past."[12]

And Tom Billings, who writes the Beyond Veg website, says, "Further, if the motivation for your diet is moral and/or spiritual, then you will want the basis of your diet to be honest as well as compassionate. In that case, ditching the false myths of naturalness presents no problems; indeed, ditching false myths means that you are ditching a burden."[13]

We agree that it just doesn't matter whether a vegan diet is our historical way of eating or not. The fact is, it makes sense *now* to choose a vegan diet. And whose diet is really natural, anyway? The assumption that there is one natural prehistoric diet, which can be approximated today and would be optimal for modern humans, is dubious at best.

Today's commercial plant foods and meats are different from the foods available in prehistoric times. We eat hybrids of plants and we feed foods to animals that they would not normally eat. Additionally, the U.S. food supply is routinely fortified with a host of vitamins and minerals. Even those people who strive to eat a more "natural" diet as adults have normally benefited from fortified foods as children. It is quite unlikely that anyone is eating a natural diet in today's world.

Taking a daily vitamin B_{12} supplement is a small thing that can make all the difference in your health as a vegan. Based on our current knowledge of vitamin B_{12} requirements and sources, supplementation is not a subject for debate. Vitamin B_{12} supplements or fortified foods are an essential part of a well-balanced and responsible vegan diet at all stages of the life cycle.

CHAPTER 4

CALCIUM, VITAMIN D, AND BONE HEALTH

CALCIUM

For most of human history, people got their calcium from plants, primarily wild, leafy greens. Dairy foods didn't become part of the human diet until around 10,000 years ago and even then they were consumed only in some parts of the world. Calcium-rich greens were so abundant in early diets that some nutritional anthropologists speculate that people consumed as much as 3,000 milligrams per day of calcium from these foods, or about three times our current recommended intakes.[1] The cultivated greens that are available to vegans today are lower in calcium than the wild vegetables available to our ancestors, but they can still make a significant contribution to calcium intake. Vegans can also get calcium from some legumes and nuts, and from fortified foods.

There is no question about whether vegan diets can provide enough calcium. They can. But that doesn't mean that they do. In studies of vegans, average calcium intakes often fall well below recommendations.[2] One unanswered question has to do with calcium needs of people who eat plant-based diets. Do vegans need less calcium? You'll see that it's not so easy to figure this out.

Calcium and Bones

While bones might seem solid and static, they are actually quite dynamic. The skeleton acts as calcium storage, providing a steady supply of calcium to the blood where it is needed for muscle relaxation, nerve cell transmission, and a host of other functions. Some of this calcium is regularly lost in the urine and must be replaced by dietary sources. As a result, bones are in motion—breaking down to release calcium to the blood and then taking up new calcium and rebuilding. Getting enough calcium is important for bone health, but reducing the amount that is lost through the urine could be important too.

Bones grow through the first three decades of life, becoming longer, heavier, and denser. By their late twenties or early thirties, most people have achieved *peak bone mass*, and their skeleton is as heavy and dense as it is going to get. There is some evidence that peak bone mass determines bone health and risk for osteoporosis in later years.

Beginning at age forty-five or so, there is a shift in metabolism and bone mass begins to decline. Efforts to slow calcium losses from the body and provide enough calcium to keep bones strong are important for preventing osteoporosis, especially for women, who can begin to lose bone rapidly after menopause.

Good bone health depends on a complex interplay of factors that affect both absorption of calcium and calcium losses from the body. Diet, lifestyle, and genetics all play a part in calcium balance. Figuring out how these factors interact and affect calcium needs has been an ongoing subject of debate among researchers, and some of the issues may be especially important for vegans.

The Relationship of Calcium Intake to Bone Health

Calcium is different from other nutrients in that it isn't associated with an acute deficiency disease. With most nutrients, if your intake is too low, you'll get sick. That's not true for calcium because levels in the blood are very tightly controlled. Even a small change in those levels can be life-threatening, so the body utilizes stored calcium in the bone plus the filtering system of the kidneys to keep calcium concentrations within strict boundaries. You can't ascertain calcium status by measuring blood levels of this mineral because those levels are always the same. But while a low calcium diet doesn't cause an acute nutritional deficiency, a chronically low intake can raise the risk for osteoporosis later in life.

Osteoporosis is a crippling and debilitating disease of severe bone loss—as much as 30 to 40 percent of total bone—that affects an estimated 10 million Americans. Eighty percent of Americans with osteoporosis are women.

When nutrition scientists look at the relationship of diet to bone health, they look at both bone density and fracture rates. And the findings are anything but clear. How much calcium humans need and the extent to which varying intakes affect bone health are topics of intense research. Many large epidemiologic studies fail to show that high calcium intakes protect against bone fractures.[3,4] The balance of evidence suggests, however, that calcium and vitamin D together are protective.[5]

Protein and Calcium: More Questions than Answers

A couple of decades ago, studies of bone health among people in different countries revealed an interesting pattern. Rates of hip fracture (which is often used as a marker for bone health) were highest in countries with the highest intakes of animal protein, even though calcium intake was also high.[6] The findings suggested that too much protein was worse for bones than too little calcium. And, in fact, there is a biological explanation to back this.

High intakes of certain proteins increase the blood's acidity, kicking off a chain of reactions to bring blood back to a more neutral pH. A release of calcium from the bones is one part of the process. The more acidic the blood, the greater the loss of calcium from bones. Meat proteins are among the most acid-producing foods, followed by proteins from grains and dairy. Diets high in fruits and vegetables are the least acidic.

Based on this, it seems to make sense that people who eat animal protein should need more calcium to replace what is constantly being leached from their bones. Conversely, wouldn't vegans, whose diets contain no animal proteins, have lower calcium needs? This sounds like an obvious conclusion, but it's not quite that straightforward.

First, the studies comparing different populations have limited use-fulness. These are ecological studies, and we saw in Chapter 1 that they provide only weak evidence. There are just too many cultural and ge-netic variations among people of Asian, African, and Caucasian back-grounds for us to make direct comparisons about their protein intakes and bone health. For example, people of African descent have a genetic predisposition toward stronger, heavier bones.[7] And a slight genetic ad-vantage in hip anatomy among Asians protects against fracture.[8]

There are cultural differences too. Asians tend to have better bal-ance, so they are less likely to fall and break a bone. And in some cul-tures, elderly people rarely leave their home without a younger family member at their side and are therefore less likely to fall. In fact, while Asian populations fare well in comparisons of hip-fracture rates, their spinal bone health is similar to westerners'.[9] This suggests that there is something in their genes or lifestyle that is specifically protective against hip fracture but doesn't affect other parts of the skeleton. If diet were the protective factor, the benefits would show up in all parts of the skeleton.

As a result, these cross-cultural studies might tell us more about culture and genetics than about diet, which means that these compar-isons don't tell us a whole lot about how much calcium western veg-ans might need.

It's better to look at clinical research, where the effects of protein are directly observed and measured. Findings from clinical studies show the following:

- Consuming *isolated animal proteins*—that is, just the pure protein portion of a food—has a direct and significant effect on calcium losses, but that effect is often lost when subjects are fed whole, high-protein foods. The reason may be that other factors in foods, like phosphorus, counteract the urinary losses.[10]
- While protein can increase calcium losses, it also enhances calcium absorption from foods. There is evidence that these positive effects on absorption may outweigh or at least compensate for the negative effects of calcium loss.[11]
- In some studies, higher protein intake is actually associated with better bone health, and protein supplements can help bone fractures heal more quickly.[12,13]

The evidence suggests that effects of protein on bone health may be dependent on how much calcium is in your diet. That is, protein is beneficial in people who consume more calcium. In addition to the positive effects of protein on calcium absorption, high-protein diets improve muscle mass, which is associated with better bone health. And protein also boosts levels of compounds that may stimulate bone formation.[14]

If all of this leaves you feeling confused, you aren't alone. The complete story about protein and calcium balance is still unfolding. But based on what we know right now, it is far too simplistic to say that vegans have lower calcium needs than omnivores or that restricting protein intake improves bone health. The science of calcium, protein, and bone health is too complex and the research too conflicting to justify those conclusions.

Vegan Diets and Bone Health

Unfortunately, a number of resources for vegans in books and online suggest that calcium requirements are lower for those on plant-based diets, and it is possible that this has not served vegans well. While we don't have much information about bone health in vegans, the few available studies suggest that some vegans don't get enough calcium. In the studies that show vegan bone health to be worse than in omnivores, it is due very simply to lower calcium intakes. So far, only one study has looked at actual risk for fracture; it found that vegans had a higher chance of breaking a bone than non-vegans—but when they consumed enough calcium, their risk of fractures was the same as in omnivores.[15]

So where does this leave us in terms of calcium requirements? Given all of the inconsistencies in the research and the findings, limited as they are, about bone health in vegans, we recommend that vegans meet the calcium recommendations that have been established for the general population.

Recommendations for daily calcium intake for western populations range from 700 milligrams in the United Kingdom to 1,000 milligrams in the United States. The U.S. recommendation is an AI, which you may remember from Chapter 1 is a "best guess" kind of recommendation. There is evidence to suggest that 700 milligrams may meet the needs of most people, but it also may not be enough for everyone. Calcium needs can vary considerably among individuals, primarily because there is a big genetic variation in absorption rates. Aiming for the U.S. recommendation of 1,000 milligrams for adults can provide good insurance.

Calcium without Milk?

Getting calcium from plants might seem a little strange in a society that is so focused on dairy foods as a source of calcium. But some research suggests that even omnivores get as much as 40 percent of their calcium from plant foods. And really, why should that be surprising? Omnivores eat broccoli, baked beans, hummus, and other plant foods that are good sources of calcium.

While a strong dairy lobby has convinced many consumers that milk and other dairy foods are essential for a healthy diet, the ability to drink milk into adulthood is not the norm throughout the world. Normal development throughout most of the world involves a gradual loss of the enzyme needed to digest milk sugar after children are weaned from breast milk. Indications are that a mutation occurred some ten centuries ago among northern Europeans that resulted in the continued production of this enzyme, allowing that population to drink milk into adulthood.

In the United States, we refer to the lack of this enzyme as "lactose intolerance." But that's definitely a western bias since this "intolerance" is not a lack or an abnormality; it's part of normal human development in most people. Since many people the world over need to meet calcium needs without dairy foods, there is no reason why vegans can't do it as well. And with our access to a wide variety of calcium-rich and fortified foods, it's not at all difficult.

Meeting Calcium Needs on a Vegan Diet

The amount of any nutrient in a food is not equal to the amount that actually makes its way from the intestines into the bloodstream. The bioavailability of a nutrient from a particular food refers to the amount of that nutrient that is likely to be absorbed and used, and it's affected by a number of factors.

A few leafy green vegetables—spinach, beet greens, Swiss chard, and rhubarb—are high in naturally occurring compounds called oxalates that bind calcium and make it essentially unavailable to the body. But the availability of calcium from low-oxalate vegetables—kale, collards, broccoli, and turnip greens—can be as high as 50 percent.[16] Calcium absorption from soyfoods, like calcium-set tofu (tofu that is processed with calcium-sulfate) and fortified soymilk, is around 25 to 30 percent, which is about the same as from cow's milk. Calcium absorption from nuts and legumes is somewhat lower, around 20 percent.

The recommended intake of 1,000 milligrams of calcium is based on the assumption that most people absorb around 30 percent of the calcium in their diet. If you're eating a varied diet that includes several different types of calcium sources, including leafy greens and soy products, you don't need to worry that some of the calcium from other foods is absorbed less efficiently.

It's possible to get plenty of calcium just from eating foods that are naturally rich in this mineral, but it does take some effort. (This is equally true for people who consume dairy foods, since many people who drink milk don't meet calcium requirements. That's why so many products on the market—from cereals to juices to protein bars—are fortified with calcium.) Using fortified foods like juices and nondairy milks can make it easier to meet calcium recommendations on a vegan diet.

It's also helpful to pay attention to the effects of processing. For example, frozen leafy greens are higher in calcium than fresh, although this is simply because their volume tends to be more concentrated. Processing also affects the amount of calcium in different types of tofu. Tofu production involves ingredients that cause soymilk to curdle. The two most common—often used together—are magnesium-chloride (*nigari* in Japanese) and calcium-sulfate. When calcium-sulfate is used, tofu is often an excellent source of calcium. Also, firm tofu tends to have a higher calcium content than soft. It's important to read package labels, though, since the amount of calcium in different brands and different types of tofu varies widely.

In the Vegan Food Guide in Chapter 7, we recommend 6 to 8 servings of calcium-rich foods per day. This allows you to mix and match small servings of a variety of calcium-rich foods or get all of your calcium from larger amounts of just a few foods. One serving is ½ cup fortified plant milk or juice, ½ cup cooked, calcium-rich vegetables, ½ cup tofu or tempeh, 2 tablespoons almond butter or tahini, ¼ cup soynuts, or ½ cup dried figs. The table on page 45 shows calcium contents of a wide variety of plant foods.

CALCIUM CONTENT OF
PLANT FOODS IN MILLIGRAMS

Food	Calcium Content (in milligrams)
Legumes (½ cup cooked)	
Black beans	51
Chickpeas	40
Great northern beans	60
Kidney beans	25
Lentils	19
Lima beans	16
Navy beans	63
Pinto beans	40
Vegetarian baked beans	43
Tofu (½ cup)	
Firm, prepared with calcium sulfate	150–300
Firm, prepared with calcium sulfate plus nigari (magnesium chloride)	100–150
Regular, prepared with calcium sulfate and nigari	100
Soft, prepared with calcium sulfate and nigari	60
Soft , prepared with nigari	30
Other soyfoods	
Soybeans, ½ cup cooked	87
Tempeh, 3½ ounces	55
TVP, ½ cup cooked	85
Soymilk, 1 cup fortified	250–300
Soymilk, 1 cup unfortified	61
Soynuts, ¼ cup	60
Nuts and seeds (2 tablespoons)	
Almonds	24
Almond butter	86
Brazil nuts	15
Sesame seeds	140
Sesame tahini	128

continues

continued

CALCIUM CONTENT OF PLANT FOODS IN MILLIGRAMS

Food	Calcium Content (in milligrams)
Vegetables (½ cup cooked)	
Bok choy	79
Broccoli, fresh	31
Broccoli, frozen	43
Butternut squash	23
Collard greens, fresh	133
Kale, fresh	47
Kale, frozen	90
Mustard greens, fresh	52
Mustard greens, frozen	76
Sweet potato	45
Turnip greens, fresh	98
Turnip greens, frozen	125
Fruits	
Dried figs, 1 cup	241
Orange, 1 medium	60
Raisins, ½ cup	41
Orange juice, calcium-fortified, 1 cup	300
Other foods	
Blackstrap molasses, 1 tablespoon	80
Corn tortilla, 6-inch	50
English muffin, made with calcium propionate	92
Fortified almond or rice milk, 1 cup	300
Quinoa, ½ cup cooked	16

Tips for Getting Enough Calcium

- Follow the recommendations in the Vegan Food Guide in Chapter 7.
- If you use calcium-fortified soymilk, give the carton a good shake before pouring since the calcium can settle to the bottom.

- Look for calcium-set tofu, which is tofu that includes calcium-sulfate as an ingredient.
- Learn to love greens! The ones that are low in oxalates—collards, kale, turnip, and mustard greens—are good sources of well-absorbed calcium as well as other nutrients that are important for bone health.
- Make your own trail mix using soynuts, almonds, and chopped figs and keep it on hand for snacks.
- Choose calcium-fortified brands when you drink fruit juices.
- If your intake falls short, make up the difference with a supplement.

VITAMIN D

Adequate vitamin D is every bit as important as calcium for maintaining bone health. But is vitamin D a nutrient? Not exactly, since we can make all we need when our skin is exposed to ultraviolet rays from sunlight. In fact, for most of human history, this is where people got their vitamin D since it occurs naturally in very few foods. But as people moved away from the equatorial zones and began to spend more time indoors, vitamin D deficiency became a problem. In the early 1900s, rickets (soft bones that don't develop well in children) was a significant public health problem that led to fortification of cow's milk with vitamin D.

While the focus has long been on bone health, more recent research suggests that suboptimal vitamin D levels are linked to fibromyalgia, rheumatoid arthritis, multiple sclerosis, depression, muscle weakness, diabetes, hypertension, and cancer. The current AI for vitamin D in adults is 600 IUs (vitamin D is also measured in micrograms; 1 microgram equals 40 IUs). But many experts believe that it may take as much as 1,000 IUs or 25 micrograms to maintain ideal blood levels of vitamin D.[17] While this continues to be a controversial area, we favor the higher recommendation.

Dietary Sources of Vitamin D

The only significant, natural sources of vitamin D in foods are fatty fish, eggs from chickens who have been fed vitamin D, and mushrooms treated with ultraviolet rays. Many people think that milk is a good natural source of vitamin D, but it isn't. Milk contains no vitamin D unless it has been fortified and is no more natural a source of this vitamin than any other fortified food.

There are two types of vitamin D used in fortified foods and supplements. Vitamin D_3 or *cholecalciferol* is derived from animals, usually from sheep's wool or fish oil. Vitamin D_2 or *ergocalciferol* is usually obtained from yeast and is vegan. The evidence suggests that the two types are absorbed equally as well but that blood levels of vitamin D_2 decline more quickly when megadoses of the vitamin are consumed.[18,19] At the smaller dose that we recommend—1,000 milligrams per day—vitamin D_2 appears to be as effective as vitamin D_3.

Getting Enough Vitamin D for Optimal Health

Concern about skin cancer has people using powerful sunscreen or shying away from sun exposure altogether. However, in addition to blocking the harmful effects of the UV light on the skin, sunscreen blocks vitamin D synthesis. And there are plenty of other factors that affect vitamin D synthesis in the skin. Older people need longer exposure and so do people with dark skin. Smog can interfere with vitamin D synthesis and the farther away you are from the equator, the more sun exposure you need to make vitamin D. Some research suggests that Americans living in the northern part of the country do not make any vitamin D during the winter months.[20]

To make adequate vitamin D for one day, a light-skinned person needs ten to fifteen minutes of midday (10:00 a.m. to 2:00 p.m.) sun exposure, without sunscreen, on a day when sunburn is possible.[21] Dark-skinned people need twenty minutes and older people need thirty minutes.[22,23]

If your sun exposure doesn't match these guidelines, then you need to take a supplement or use fortified foods. We recommend 25 micrograms (1,000 IU) per day of vitamin D_2.

Many foods, including most breakfast cereals, are fortified with vitamin D. Almost all use vitamin D_3, which is derived from animals. Most brands of fortified soymilk and other nondairy milks use vitamin D_2, which comes from yeast exposed to UV rays.

For food labeling purposes, the Daily Value for vitamin D is 10 micrograms (400 IU). So if a food provides 25 percent of the Daily Value for vitamin D, it contains 2.5 micrograms (100 IU) of vitamin D per serving. Vitamin D–fortified soy, almond, hemp, or rice milk normally has 2 to 3 micrograms (80 to 120 IU) per cup. You can see from these numbers that it's not that easy to meet the recommended 1,000 IU per day from fortified foods. If your sun exposure isn't adequate, you will probably need to use a vitamin D supplement. Most natural foods stores carry supplements of plant-derived vitamin D_2, or you can order one from the online sources in the resource section of this book.

Bone Health: More than Calcium and Vitamin D

Calcium and vitamin D have well-deserved reputations as bone-strengthening nutrients, but they don't act alone. The following are all important for protecting bone health.

- Stay physically active. Exercise is absolutely crucial to bone density and strength; it's probably the single most important factor in preventing bone loss. Choose weight-bearing and high-impact exercise to get the greatest benefit, such as weight-lifting, jogging, and step aerobics. Biking and swimming are not especially valuable to strengthening bones.
- Maintain a healthy weight and by this, we mean don't let your weight get too low. When it comes to bone health, being a few pounds above your ideal weight is better than being a few pounds below it. Rapid weight loss is associated with bone loss, so if you

have some pounds to shed, aim for a slow reduction while building more muscle and protecting bones through exercise.

- Eat plenty of fruits and vegetables because they keep the blood more alkaline. In fact, some researchers have suggested that the best diet for maintaining healthy bones is one that is rich in calcium, contains plenty of protein to boost calcium absorption, and is generous in fruits and vegetables to keep the blood alkaline. But fruits and vegetables also provide nutrients that are good for bones, such as vitamin K and the minerals boron, potassium, and magnesium. Vitamin C also plays a role in bone formation and high vitamin C intake has been linked to better bone health. Plant foods are the best sources of vitamin K and potassium, and they are the only sources of vitamin C.

- Avoid excess sodium, which is linked to calcium losses. Lightly salting your food is fine, but an overdependence on processed foods can make vegan diets too high in sodium.

 Building Healthy Bones on a Vegan Diet

Building and keeping strong bones depends on a number of lifestyle factors. They are all important.

- Aim for a diet that is rich in calcium, using the tips for meeting calcium needs on pages 46–47.
- Eat a protein-rich diet by following the guidelines in Chapter 7.
- Include plenty of vegetables and fruits in your diet.
- Get adequate sun exposure to make vitamin D or take a supplement that provides 25 micrograms (1,000 IU) per day.
- Stay active and include weight-bearing exercise in your fitness routine.
- Avoid excess sodium.

CHAPTER 5

FATS
Making the Best Choices

S tudies show that, on average, vegans consume a little less than 30 percent of their calories from fat. That's a bit lower than the average for non-vegan Americans, but not by much. The big difference is in the type of fat that vegans consume since plant foods are much lower in saturated fat than meat, dairy, and eggs.

The term "fat" is a big category that includes a number of different fatty acids, two of which are essential to our diet. Actual requirements for essential fats are low, but there may be advantages to eating some fat-rich foods overall. In this chapter, we'll look at three issues: the long-chain omega-3 fats, meeting essential fatty acid needs, and the question of how much fat vegans can safely consume.

LONG-CHAIN OMEGA 3 FATS

EPA and DHA are the "long-chain" omega-3 fatty acids that are found mainly in cold water fish. These fats are thought to be important for cardiovascular disease primarily because they reduce blood clotting and inflammation.[1] Because DHA is found in nerve tissue, inadequate levels could also be linked to neurological problems such as dementia and depression.[2,3]

Since the long-chain omega-3 fats are found primarily in fish and to a much smaller extent in eggs, lacto-ovo vegetarians consume very little, and vegans generally have none in their diets (although some

Dietary Fats: Terms You Need to Know

The Essential Fatty Acids
   Linoleic Acid (LA): An omega-6 fatty acid found in grains, seeds, nuts, and oils, especially safflower, sunflower, corn, and soy oil.
   Alpha-Linolenic Acid (ALA): A short-chain omega-3 fatty acid found in flaxseeds, chia seeds, hemp seeds, walnuts, canola oil, and some soyfoods.

Long-Chain Omega-3 Fats
   DHA (docosahexanoic acid): Found in fatty fish, some eggs, and algae. It can be manufactured in the body from ALA, but optimal conditions for conversion are not well-known.
   EPA (eicosapentanoic acid): Found in fatty fish, sea vegetables, and algae. It can be manufactured in the body from ALA, and small amounts can be made from DHA.

vegans may consume very small amounts of EPA from sea vegetables).[4] Whether or not this matters is a big question in vegan nutrition.

Potential Benefits of DHA and EPA:
The Science behind the Claims

A number of studies (and large reviews of studies) have suggested that omega-3 fats reduce the risk of heart disease, but others have found no benefit. There has been so much published on this subject that it makes it almost impossible to analyze the individual studies. We need to rely on systematic reviews and meta-analyses instead. But even the reviews have been conflicting; two large ones published in 2006 reached opposite conclusions. When research is this inconsistent, it probably indicates that the benefits are modest at best.

Although the omega-3 blood levels of vegetarians have been measured often enough to show that they are clearly lower than in fish-eaters, the actual effects of these lower levels aren't clear. A 1999 study in Chile found that vegetarians had significantly more platelets (which are involved in blood clotting) and a shorter bleeding time than non-vegetarians.[5] This suggests greater blood-clotting activity, which could raise heart disease risk. But when the vegetarians were supplemented with EPA and DHA for eight weeks, the bleeding time stayed the same (although other factors changed).[6]

In a 1992 study in the United Kingdom, there were only small differences between vegetarians and non-vegetarians in factors that affect blood clotting, and bleeding times were similar.[7]

So, of two studies looking at these effects, vegetarians fared worse than meat-eaters in one but were largely the same in the other. We need a lot more information before we can draw firm conclusions. Whether these lower omega-3 intakes increase risk in vegetarians for autoimmune diseases (which are affected by inflammation) or depression or dementia hasn't been studied, but right now there is no strong evidence that they do. And people who eat seafood but not other meat don't appear to be at lower risk for death from heart disease than vegetarians.[8]

OMEGA-3 FATS IN PLANTS

While plant foods don't have DHA and EPA, a few provide alpha-linolenic acid (ALA). This is a short-chain omega-3 fat that is essential in diets and technically can be converted to EPA and DHA. It's found in flaxseeds, hempseeds, chia seeds, canola oil, walnuts, soy oil, and some soyfoods.

A second fatty acid called linoleic acid (LA) is also essential in the diet. This is an omega-6 fat and it's abundant in commonly consumed oils like safflower and sunflower oil as well as whole plant foods. Americans, including vegans, get plenty of this essential fat.

The problem is that high intakes of the omega-6 fatty acid LA suppress conversion of ALA to DHA and EPA. Experts suggest that for optimal production of DHA and EPA, diets should contain no more than a 4 to 1 ratio of LA to ALA. But the ratio in vegan diets is more typically around 15 to 1.[9] That is, vegans are consuming too much of the omega-6 fatty acid LA and sometimes not getting enough of the omega-3 fat ALA. As a result, dietary strategies to boost ALA intake and lower LA intake have become popular among some vegans. But do they work?

Unfortunately, there are no long-term studies looking at blood levels of EPA and DHA in vegetarians when these strategies are used. And short-term studies indicate that it takes large amounts of ALA to increase the amount of DHA in the blood. In fact, for the most part, studies using supplements or food sources of ALA have been largely unsuccessful in raising levels of DHA and only moderately successful in raising levels of EPA.

In addition, it's not clear that high doses of the short-chain omega-3s are completely benign. In the Nurses' Health Study, higher intakes of ALA were linked to eye problems, including increased risk of macular degeneration.[10] In contrast, the highest intakes of DHA tended to be protective of eye health. These studies were done on only one population by one group of researchers, and the biggest contributors of ALA in omnivore diets are dairy and other animal products, not plant foods. So it's not clear whether these findings are relevant to vegans. The findings suggest caution regarding high intakes of ALA, but more information is needed before we should draw conclusions.

Based on the little we know, it's not clear that large amounts of ALA are safe. Nor is it clear that increasing ALA intake boosts blood levels of DHA and EPA. But there is another option for vegans: algae-derived DHA and EPA supplements.

DHA SUPPLEMENTS

Fish get their DHA from algae, and vegans can go to the same source. Preliminary research suggests that a supplement providing 200 milligrams of DHA per day for three months can raise blood DHA levels in vegans by as much as 50 percent.[11] Other studies of vegetarians (not necessarily vegans) have also shown the positive effects of taking DHA supplements.[12]

But because the research on the overall benefits of omega-3s is so conflicting, it's hard to know whether these supplements are useful for vegans. We are not convinced that they are. On the other hand, we are not convinced that the lower blood levels of DHA and EPA in vegans is unimportant. Until we know more, we are inclined to recommend supplementing with very small amounts, around 200 to 300 milligrams of DHA (or DHA and EPA combined), every two or three days.

Many vegan supplements provide only DHA, but new ones providing both DHA and EPA are becoming available. A few vegan foods such as soymilk, energy bars, and olive oil are also fortified with algae-derived DHA.

MEETING ESSENTIAL FATTY ACID NEEDS

While large intakes may not be advisable, everyone needs to consume some ALA since it's an essential fatty acid. Recommended intakes of ALA for adults are 1.1 grams per day for women and 1.6 grams for men. Meeting those needs isn't difficult, but it requires a little bit of attention since ALA is not widely available in foods.

Each of the following provides around one-quarter of the daily ALA requirement for an adult male or one-third the requirement for an adult female. To meet the ALA needs of an adult woman, choose three servings from these foods, and for an adult man, choose four.

1 teaspoon canola oil
¼ teaspoon flaxseed oil (just a few drops)
⅔ teaspoon hempseed oil
1 teaspoon walnut oil
2 teaspoons ground English walnuts or 1 walnut half
1 teaspoon ground flaxseeds*
½ cup cooked soybeans

*Don't use whole flaxseeds since they aren't well-digested and the ALA is poorly absorbed.

1 cup firm tofu
1 cup tempeh
2 tablespoons soynuts

HOW MUCH FAT SHOULD VEGANS CONSUME?

Despite the popularity of vegan diets that eliminate all high-fat foods, there hasn't been much research comparing very low-fat vegan diets to those that include some higher-fat plant foods. And there is reason to think that very low-fat vegan diets are not ideal. Eating diets that are too low in fat could be the reason that some people abandon vegan diets and return to eating meat. Many think of meat as "protein," forgetting that these foods are also typically high in fat. People who don't feel well on vegan diets sometimes add meat back to their diet because they're convinced that they aren't getting adequate protein—when, in fact, they might have felt better by simply adding more fat to their menu.

Contrary to popular opinion, diets that include fat from plant foods are not linked to heart disease. (We'll talk more about this in Chapter 13.) And the idea that high-fat diets are linked to cancer risk is weak. Most importantly, plant foods that are naturally high in fat are beneficial to health. There is a large body of research showing that nuts protect against heart disease. They are also rich in vitamins, minerals, and phytochemicals. You'll see in Chapter 7 that we recommend that all vegans include a serving or two of nuts in their meals every day.

Higher fat foods can also make it easier for vegan children to meet calorie needs. And while it's somewhat of a paradox, we'll see in Chapter 13 that including some of these foods in weight-reduction diets can improve success.

These foods make vegan diets more interesting and easier to plan, which means that they make it more realistic for people to transition to a vegan diet and stick with it for the long-term. From both a practical and a health point of view, it doesn't make sense to ban high-fat foods from vegan diets. And as we'll see below, even oils can play a role in healthy vegan diets.

Fat in Vegan Diets: Practical Guidelines

- **Keep total fat intake in the moderate range.** There is no consensus of opinion among experts on the ideal level of fat in the diet. Excessive fat intake is not healthy, but that doesn't mean that all fat is bad. The World Health Organization cautions against consuming a diet that is less than 15 percent fat for adults or less than 20 percent for premenopausal women.[13] We recommend that vegans strive for a fat intake somewhere between 20 and 30 percent of calories. That means between 22 and 33 grams of fat for every 1,000 calories you consume. Here is a quick guide to approximate amounts of fat in plant foods:

Food	Average Amount of Fat (in grams)
Avocado, ¼ cup cubes	5.5
Leafy green vegetables, ½ cup cooked	0.2–0.35
Nuts, ¼ cup	17–20
Seeds, 2 tablespoons	8
Soybeans, ½ cup cooked	7
Tempeh, ½ cup	9
Tofu, firm, ½ cup	11
Tofu, soft, ½ cup	4.5
Vegetable oils, 1 teaspoon	5

- **Avoid fats that are associated with chronic disease risk.** We'll talk more about these in Chapter 13, but both saturated fat and trans fats may raise the risk for heart disease and diabetes and could be associated with cancer risk as well. Generally speaking, vegans don't need to worry since both tend to be low in plant-based diets. Watch for labels that include "partially hydrogenated vegetable oil," a type of fat that is high in trans fats.
- **Limit intake of oils high in the omega-6 fat linoleic acid.** These include corn, soy, safflower, sunflower, and to a lesser extent, peanut

and sesame oils. Watch for prepared foods that include these oils toward the top of the ingredient list.

- **Get most of your fat from foods that provide monounsaturated fat.** Best sources are nuts, nut butters, avocados, and olives, and olive, canola, or high-oleic safflower and sunflower oils.
- **Be sure to meet your needs for the essential omega-3 fatty acid ALA.** Follow the guidelines on page 55 to make sure you're getting enough of this fat.
- **Consider taking a DHA supplement.** Vegans over the age of sixty, especially, should consider taking a DHA (or DHA plus EPA) supplement of 200 to 300 milligrams a day. Younger vegans might consider taking this much every two to three days.

VEGETABLE OILS IN VEGAN DIETS

You don't have to include vegetable oils in your diet, but they can fit into a healthy vegan eating plan. Not all vegetable oils are equal, though. Since vegans tend to have a high ratio of LA to ALA in their diets, it's a good idea to choose oils that are low in LA. Another consideration is the smoke point of oils. Oils with a low smoke point begin to break down at high temperatures, producing potentially toxic compounds. Smoke point is affected by the type of fatty acids in the oil as well as processing. Oils with a higher monounsaturated fat content have a higher smoke point, which makes them better for cooking. Cold-pressed or unrefined oils have a higher percentage of protective phytochemicals, but they also have a lower smoke point, so they are better to use in dressings than for cooking.

For baking and cooking, choose these oils most often:

- Extra virgin olive oil: All types of olive oil are high in monounsaturated fats, but extra virgin olive oil also contains compounds that may protect against heart disease, cancer, and stroke. Its smoke point is only moderately high, so use it only for sautéing foods at lower temperatures or for cold or warm salads.

- Canola oil: It is high in monounsaturated fats and has a some-what higher smoke point than olive oil.
- High-oleic sunflower or safflower oils: These are special hybrids grown to produce an oil that is rich in monounsaturated fat. They must say "high oleic" on the label.
- Almond, avocado, hazelnut, and macadamia nut oils: These are all rich in monounsaturated fats, and their high smoke points make them a good choice for cooking. They tend to be expensive, but you may want to splurge on them occasionally for special dishes.

Minimize these oils in your diet:

- Corn, soybean, safflower, and sunflower oils (unless labeled as "high oleic"). These are popular for frying because they have high smoke points. But all are high in the omega-6 fatty acid linoleic acid (LA) and should be minimized in the diet. Anything labeled "vegetable oil" is almost always soybean oil.
- Peanut and sesame oils: These are moderately high in mono-unsaturated fats and have a relatively high smoke point, but both—particularly sesame oil—have a fairly high LA content.

Use these oils only as supplements:

- Flaxseed and hempseed oils: Because of their very high ALA content (especially for flaxseed), these oils are generally used in small quantities as a supplement—perhaps sprinkled over vegeta-bles. They have low smoke points and should never be heated.

WHAT ABOUT COCONUT OIL?

Packed with saturated fat—it has more than either butter or lard—coconut oil has developed a surprising reputation as a health food. This is partly because some research has shown coconut oil to have anti-microbial properties. Also, the main fat in coconut oil, which is called lauric acid, raises good HDL cholesterol, producing a favorable cholesterol profile. Virgin coconut oil contains a number of protective phytochemicals as well and, for people eating healthy diets containing plenty of fiber-rich plant foods, coconut oil consumption isn't associated with heart disease. Cooks may like it for its appealing flavor as well as the fact that it is particularly stable and doesn't turn rancid easily. It can also be useful when you need a solid fat for cooking. But the jury is still out on the health effects of coconut oil, so, like all added fats, it should be used in moderation.

CHAPTER 6

IRON, ZINC, IODINE, AND VITAMIN A
Maximizing Vegan Sources

Protein, calcium, and vitamins B_{12} and D get most of the attention in vegan diets. But there is a handful of other nutrients that deserve consideration, namely iron, zinc, iodine, and vitamin A. We'll touch briefly on vitamin K, riboflavin, potassium, and selenium too.

MINERAL ABSORPTION ON VEGAN DIETS

Minerals like iron and zinc are absorbed less well from plant foods than from animal products. There are a number of reasons for this, but the most important is the presence of phytate in the diet. This phosphorus-containing compound is found in whole grains, legumes, seeds, and nuts. (Smaller amounts are found in vegetables too.) Phytate binds minerals, making them less absorbable. Refining grains reduces their phytate content, but it also reduces the mineral content of a food, so isn't much of a solution.

A number of food preparation techniques help liberate minerals from phytate and can greatly increase absorption. Fermentation, which includes the activity of both yeast and sourdough starters in bread making, as well as the production of fermented foods like tempeh and miso, greatly increases mineral availability. This makes leavened bread a better source of well-absorbed iron and zinc than crackers and flat breads.

The addition of citrus fruits to meals can also boost mineral absorption. Foods that contain vitamin C are especially effective for increasing iron absorption. Toasting nuts and seeds, and sprouting beans and grains, reduces the effects of phytate. So does soaking these foods and discarding the water before using them in a recipe.

Phytate isn't all bad, though. It's an antioxidant that acts in ways that could reduce cancer risk. This suggests a benefit to getting minerals from plant foods. If you use food preparation techniques to break the bond between phytate and iron or zinc, you'll improve mineral absorption while getting the potential health benefits of phytate.

IRON

You might be surprised to know that vegans typically consume more iron than either lacto-ovo vegetarians or meat-eaters.[1] The issue for vegans is how well that iron is absorbed.

This essential mineral is a part of hemoglobin, the component of red blood cells that is needed to ferry oxygen to the cells. It's also a part of many enzymes involved in energy production and immune function. Even among Americans who eat meat, iron deficiency is the most common nutrient deficiency.

We need a constant supply of iron in our diets because we lose it through daily sloughing off of intestinal and other cells. Premenopausal women lose more iron than men because of menstrual losses. Therefore, their iron needs are more than twice what men require. The recommended daily iron intake is 18 milligrams for premenopausal women and 8 milligrams for men and postmenopausal women. In the government's ongoing survey of American eating habits, 12 percent of women between the ages of twelve and forty-nine had poor iron status.[2]

Iron Deficiency

There are two stages of iron deficiency. In the first, iron stores become depleted and there may be a decrease in hemoglobin levels and mild symptoms. In the next stage—overt iron deficiency anemia—hemoglobin drops to subnormal levels, which can cause symptoms such as pale skin, fatigue, weakness, shortness of breath, an inability to maintain body temperature, loss of appetite, and hair loss. But these symptoms can also be due to other nutritional deficiencies or conditions, and true iron-deficiency anemia can be diagnosed only through a blood test. It's relatively inexpensive to have your iron levels tested by a doctor. A blood test can also help your physician differentiate between anemia due to iron deficiency and anemia due to vitamin B_{12} deficiency.

Meat Iron versus Plant Iron

Foods contain two forms of iron, called heme and nonheme iron. Heme iron is much more readily absorbed by the body and is not much affected by other factors in the diet. Nonheme iron is absorbed at a much lower level, and its absorption can be inhibited or enhanced by other dietary components. Meat contains both types of iron, but plant foods contain only nonheme iron. So using strategies to boost absorption is important for people who get all of their iron from plant foods.

Because phytate reduces iron absorption, all of the food preparation methods we mentioned above—fermentation, leavening breads, soaking, sprouting, and cooking—can boost iron absorption. But the most effective way by far to release iron from phytate is to add vitamin C to meals. The effects of vitamin C on iron absorption are rather dramatic. In one study in India, children with iron-deficiency anemia (who probably did not have high vitamin C intakes) were given 100 milligrams of vitamin C at lunch and dinner for sixty days. Most made a full recovery with a significant improvement in their anemia.[3]

But simply taking a daily vitamin C supplement won't improve your iron status, since the iron and vitamin C must be consumed at the same time. So including iron-rich and vitamin C–rich foods in the same meal is important for good iron status. Vitamin C is found in citrus fruits, strawberries, green leafy vegetables (broccoli, kale, collards, swiss chard, brussels sprouts), bell peppers (yellow, red, and green), and cauliflower.

Other organic acids in fruits and vegetables may also boost iron absorption. Cooking foods in cast-iron pans can increase iron consumption
from acidic foods like tomato sauce.

You should know, however, that certain dietary factors like tannins in coffee and tea and high doses of calcium reduce absorption of
nonheme iron. It's important to take calcium supplements between
meals and avoid drinking coffee and tea with meals to maximize iron
absorption.

Vegans have a definite advantage over lacto-ovo vegetarians when
it comes to iron because milk is a poor source of this mineral. In addition to displacing iron-rich foods from the diet, it interferes with iron
absorption. Excessive consumption of milk can increase the risk for
iron deficiency, especially in young children.[4]

Vegan and Vegetarian DRI for Iron

Vegetarians typically have iron stores that are at the lower end of the
normal range—that is, lower than the stores of meat-eaters, but still
adequate. It's important to maintain these stores by eating plenty of iron-
rich foods. And since nonheme iron is absorbed at a lower rate, vegetarians and vegans need more dietary iron than meat-eaters. But how much
more is controversial. The Institute of Medicine established a vegetarian
recommendation that is 1.8 times higher for vegetarians than omnivores. But this was based on a (completely unrealistic) test diet that was
low in vitamin C and high in factors (like tannins from tea) that reduce
iron absorption.[5] In other words, it represents a worst-case scenario
rather than the way most vegetarians and vegans actually eat.

Based on these recommendations, a premenopausal vegan woman
would require 33 milligrams of iron per day. While it's possible to plan
a diet that provides this much iron, it would be extremely difficult
to consume this much without supplements. Moreover, in addition to
being unrealistic, this amount is probably unnecessary. Vegans who
consume vitamin C–rich foods with their meals and who avoid coffee,

tea, and calcium supplements with meals are likely to need much less iron than this recommendation. See "Maximizing Iron and Zinc in Vegan Diets" on page 70.

If you are diagnosed with iron-deficiency anemia, it doesn't mean you should start eating meat. Iron deficiency, even in meat-eaters, is usually treated with supplemental iron, not more meat. Large doses of iron should be taken only under a doctor's care, however, since megadoses of any mineral can be harmful. There may also be an advantage to taking supplements of the amino acid L-lysine since, in one study of women whose iron stores were not improved with supplements, adding 1.5 to 2 grams per day of L-lysine to their diet increased their iron stores.[6]

IRON CONTENT OF VEGAN FOODS

Food	Iron Content (in milligrams)
Breads, cereals, grains	
Barley, pearled, ½ cup, cooked	1.0
Bran flakes, 1 cup	10.5
Bread, white, 1 slice	0.9
Bread, whole wheat, 1 slice	0.9
Cream of Wheat, ½ cup cooked	5.8
Oatmeal, instant, 1 packet	8.2
Pasta, enriched, ½ cup cooked	0.9
Rice, brown, ½ cup cooked	0.4
Wheat germ, 2 tablespoons	1.4
Vegetables (½ cup cooked unless otherwise indicated)	
Asparagus	0.8
Beet greens	1.4
Bok choy	0.9
Broccoli rabe	1.0
Brussels sprouts	0.9
Collard greens	1.1
Peas	1.2
Pumpkin	1.7
Spinach	3.2

continues

continued

IRON CONTENT OF VEGAN FOODS

Food	Iron Content (in milligrams)
Vegetables (continued)	
Swiss chard	2.0
Tomato juice, 1 cup	1.0
Tomato sauce	0.9
Sea vegetables (½ cup cooked)	
Dulse, dry	11.2
Kombu, dry	38.6
Nori, dry	6.5
Wakame, dry	5.8
Fruits	
Apricots, dried, ¼ cup	0.9
Prunes, ¼ cup	1.2
Prune juice, 6 ounces	2.3
Raisins, ¼ cup	0.8
Legumes (½ cup cooked)	
Black beans	1.8
Black-eyed peas	2.2
Garbanzo beans	2.4
Kidney beans	2.0
Lentils	3.3
Lima beans	2.2
Navy beans	2.3
Pinto beans	2.2
Split peas	1.3
Vegetarian baked beans	1.7
Soyfoods	
Soybeans, ½ cup cooked	4.4
Soymilk, 1 cup	1.1–1.8*
Tempeh, ½ cup	1.3
Tofu, firm, ½ cup	2.0
Textured vegetable protein, ¼ cup, dry	1.4
Veggie "meats," fortified, 1 ounce	0.8–2.1*

*Amount varies by brand.

continued

IRON CONTENT OF VEGAN FOODS

Food	Iron Content (in milligrams)
Nuts and seeds	
Almonds, ¼ cup	1.3
Almond butter, 2 tablespoons	1.1
Cashews, ¼ cup	2.0
Peanuts, ¼ cup	1.7
Peanut butter, 2 tablespoons	0.6
Pecans, ¼ cup	0.7
Pine nuts, 2 tablespoons	0.47
Pumpkin seeds, 2 tablespoons	0.25
Sunflower seeds	1.1
Tahini	0.75
Other foods	
Blackstrap molasses, 1 tablespoon	3.6
Dark chocolate, 1 ounce	3.9
Energy bar, 1 bar	1.4–4.5*

*Amount varies by brand.

ZINC

Zinc is a tricky issue for vegans—and for nutritionists. This mineral is needed for at least 100 different enzymatic reactions in the body. It's required for protein synthesis, cell growth, blood formation, and immune function. While overt zinc deficiency is rarely seen in western countries, it's possible that some people—especially children in low-income families—suffer from marginal deficiency. Poor growth in children is one sign of a marginal deficiency. But because zinc is used for so many functions, there might be other suboptimal health conditions related to low zinc intake that we don't really understand yet. It's also somewhat difficult to measure zinc status accurately.

As a result, we have some unanswered questions about zinc. And one of those questions is: How much zinc do vegans need?

Factors Affecting Zinc Requirements

The adult RDAs for zinc are 11 milligrams for men and 8 milligrams for women. Some studies show that vegans consume around 10 to 13 milligrams per day, which is slightly less zinc than omnivores—but for the most part, intakes are pretty comparable.

However, absorption from plant foods is quite a bit lower than from animal foods, and the Food and Nutrition Board suggests that zinc needs could be as much as 50 percent greater for vegans. That means that vegan zinc needs would be 16½ milligrams for men and 12 milligrams for women. While there is no evidence that vegans and other vegetarians suffer from zinc deficiency and there is evidence that they could adapt to lower absorption, it's important to optimize zinc absorption. As with iron, phytate is one of the important factors affecting zinc bioavailability, so many of the food preparation techniques that boost iron absorption also work for zinc. See "Maximizing Iron and Zinc in Vegan Diets" on page 70 for guidelines on getting enough zinc. If you think that your diet may fall short on well-absorbed zinc, consider taking a multivitamin that contains zinc. Or if you are already taking calcium tablets, choose one with zinc.

ZINC CONTENT OF FOODS

Food	Zinc Content (in milligrams)
Breads, cereals, grains	
Barley, pearled, ½ cup cooked	0.6
Bran flakes, 1 cup	2.0
Granola, ¼ cup	1.3
Millet, ½ cup cooked	0.8
Oatmeal, instant, 1 packet	1.0
Quinoa, ½ cup cooked	1.0
Rice, brown, ½ cup cooked	0.6
Wheat germ, 2 tablespoons	2.7

continues

continued

ZINC CONTENT OF FOODS

Food	Zinc Content (in milligrams)
Vegetables (½ cup cooked)	
Asparagus	0.5
Avocado, ½	0.6
Broccoli	0.4
Corn	0.5
Mushrooms	0.7
Peas	0.5
Spinach	0.7
Legumes (½ cup cooked)	
Adzuki beans	2.0
Black-eyed peas	1.1
Chickpeas	1.2
Kidney beans	0.9
Lentils	1.3
Lima beans	0.9
Navy beans	0.9
Pinto beans	0.8
Split peas	1.0
Soyfoods	
Soybeans, ½ cup cooked	1.0
Tempeh, ½ cup cooked	1.0
Tofu, firm, ½ cup	1.1
Veggie "meats," fortified, 1 ounce	1.4–1.8*
Nuts and seeds (2 tablespoons)	
Almond butter	1.0
Brazil nuts	0.7
Cashews	0.9
Peanuts	1.1
Peanut butter	0.9
Pumpkin/squash seeds	1.1
Sunflower seeds	0.9
Tahini	1.4
Other foods	
Chocolate, dark, 1 ounce	1.0
Energy bar, 1 bar	3.0–5.2*

*Amount varies by brand.

Maximizing Iron and Zinc in Vegan Diets

- Use the tables on pages 65 and 68 to make sure you're choosing plenty of foods rich in iron and zinc. Good sources of iron are beans, leafy green vegetables, sea vegetables, and dried fruit. Good sources of zinc are beans, nuts, peanuts, peanut butter, pumpkin seeds, sunflower seeds, bran flakes, wheat germ, and tempeh.
- Include a good source of vitamin C at every meal. Among the best sources are citrus fruits, broccoli, leafy green vegetables, bell peppers, strawberries, brussels sprouts, and cauliflower.
- Consume coffee and tea between meals rather than with meals.
- Take calcium supplements between meals rather than with meals.
- Toast nuts before adding them to recipes.
- If you enjoy sprouting beans and grains, this is another way to boost mineral absorption.
- Choose leavened breads and sourdough bread more often than flat breads and crackers. Refined grains like white bread have much lower amounts of phytate, and while they may be fortified with iron, they have far less zinc than whole-grain products. Even though absorption is lower from whole grains, the total amount of zinc absorbed is usually greater from whole grains.

IODINE

Most people don't give a second's thought to iodine, a mineral that is needed for healthy thyroid function. But throughout the world, iodine deficiency is a serious public health problem. Deficiency in pregnancy is especially serious since it can impact brain development in the fetus.

Eating either too much or too little iodine can cause the thyroid gland to become enlarged, which is called a goiter. When iodine intake is too low, it causes hypothyroidism, resulting in slowed metabolism, elevated cholesterol, and weight gain. Too much iodine can cause either hypothyroidism or hyperthyroidism.

In the United States, most people get enough iodine by using iodized salt or eating fish or dairy products. Milk and other dairy foods aren't necessarily good sources of iodine, but iodized solutions are used to clean the cows' teats and dairy equipment, and the iodine ends up in the milk itself. In some parts of the world, sea vegetables (seaweeds) provide iodine.

The iodine content of most plant foods is variable, though, because it depends on the iodine content of the soil. Foods grown closer to the ocean tend to be higher in iodine. (In fact, even ocean mist can provide iodine, although it's not a reliable or measurable source.) In some parts of Europe, where salt is not iodized at high enough levels (or at all) and the iodine content of plants is poor, vegans who don't use supplements could have abnormal thyroid function.[8]

Naturally occurring compounds known as goitrogens, which are found in soybeans, flax seeds, and raw cruciferous vegetables (broccoli, brussels sprouts, cauliflower, and cabbage) counteract the activity of iodine. A diet high in goitrogens can cause hypothyroidism if the diet is too low in iodine. But as long as your diet is adequate in iodine, there is no reason to avoid soyfoods or other sources of goitrogens. See Chapter 15 for more discussion on the safety of soyfoods.

Meeting Iodine Needs

The recommended iodine intake for adults is 150 micrograms per day. Vegans can get adequate iodine if they do any one of the following:

- If you add salt to your foods, use iodized salt. If you don't typically add salt to your foods, don't start doing so just to get iodine. One-quarter teaspoon provides 76 micrograms of iodine. Different "natural" salt preparations, including sea salt, have variable amounts of iodine and aren't dependable. Sea salt also has the same detrimental effects on blood pressure and bone health as regular salt. The salt added to processed and fast foods is rarely iodized.

- Consume sea vegetables like kelp, nori, dulse, and alaria several times per week. This is a tricky way to get iodine, though, since the amounts are so variable. And some sea veggies are extremely high in iodine, which can cause thyroid problems. So while consuming sea vegetables three to four times per week can be helpful, we recommend that you not eat them more often than that.
- Take a modest iodine supplement providing 75 to 150 micrograms of iodine three to four times per week. If you take a vegan multivitamin, check the label since it probably contains iodine. Using a supplement is our favorite way to get iodine since it is reliable (unlike sea vegetables) and harmless (unlike salt). Don't overdo it with supplements, though, since the range of safe iodine intake is relatively small, and it's important to avoid intakes above the upper limit for safety.

RDAs AND UPPER LIMITS FOR IODINE INTAKE

Age (years)	RDA (micrograms)	Upper Limit (micrograms)
1–3	90	200
4–8	90	300
9–13	120	600
14–18	150	900
Over 18	150	1,100
Pregnant		
18 or younger	220	900
Over 18	220	1,100
Lactating		
18 or younger	290	900
Over 18	290	1,100

VITAMIN A

The active form of vitamin A is retinol and it is found only in animal products. But plants have more than fifty compounds called carotenoids that the body can convert to vitamin A. The most common is beta-carotene. Because there are so many forms of vitamin A, the vitamin A content of foods is stated as retinol activity equivalents (RAE). Think of these as the amount of potential vitamin A activity in a food. The RDA for vitamin A is 900 RAE for men and 700 RAE for women.

In addition to their role as vitamin A precursors, the carotenoids have antioxidant properties and other potential benefits for reducing chronic disease. The preformed vitamin A in animal foods doesn't have those advantages.

In 2000, based on new evidence about the conversion of beta-carotene into active vitamin A, the FNB doubled their estimate of how much beta-carotene it takes to produce adequate vitamin A. That means that the RAE content of plant foods is only half of what was previously thought. Where we once thought that vegan diets automatically provided enough vitamin A, it's now clear that getting enough requires at least some diligence.

As you can see from the table on page 74, carrot juice is very high in vitamin A. If you like carrot juice, consider drinking ¼ cup per day to give your vitamin A intake a boost. A varied diet that includes plenty of brightly colored vegetables should make up the rest of your requirements. Both cooking and added fat increase the absorption of beta-carotene, so there is a benefit to eating some of these vegetables cooked rather than raw. And it's a good idea not to let the fat content in your meals drop too low.

VITAMIN A CONTENT OF PLANT FOODS

Recommended intake is 700 RAE for adult women and 900 RAE for adult men.

Food	Vitamin A Content (in retinol activity equivalents or RAE)
Vegetables (½ cup cooked unless otherwise indicated)	
Beet greens	276
Broccoli	60
Bok choy	180
Butternut squash	572
Carrots, 1 medium, raw	509
Carrots, ½ cup cooked	665
Carrot juice, 1 cup	2,256
Chicory greens, 1 cup raw	166
Collard greens	148
Dandelion greens	356
Hubbard squash	382
Kale	443
Mustard greens	221
Pumpkin, canned	953
Spinach	472
Sweet potatoes	961
Swiss chard	268
Tomato, 1 medium	76
Tomato juice, 1 cup	56
Fruits	
Apricots, 3 fresh (not dried)	101
Cantaloupe, 1 cup chunks	270
Mango, 1 medium	80
Nectarine, 1 medium	50
Papaya, 1 medium	167

VITAMIN K

Although vitamin K was discovered in the early part of the twentieth century, its exact function in the human body wasn't understood until 1974, which is pretty recent in the world of nutrients.

Vitamin K is essential for blood clotting, and most people get enough to support that function. But research suggests that vitamin K also contributes to bone health. Older people with higher vitamin K intakes and higher blood levels of vitamin K appear to be at lower risk for hip fracture.[9]

Because of some errors in measuring vitamin K content of foods, there is evidence now that people have lower vitamin K intakes than previously thought. This isn't an issue for blood clotting but it may be for bone health. The best sources of vitamin K are leafy green vegetables.

Soy, canola, and olive oils are also good sources. Since vitamin K is fat soluble, cooking greens in a small amount of oil can help your body absorb more.

There isn't much information about the vitamin K intake of vegetarians or vegans, but what we know suggests that people eating plant-based diets get plenty. So why have we singled it out for discussion? The answer has to do with claims that have been made about vitamin K from those who question the adequacy of vegan diets.

The term "vitamin K" actually refers to two slightly different compounds with vitamin K activity. One, called phylloquinone or vitamin K_1, is found in both plant and animal foods. The other, menaquinone or vitamin K_2, is produced by bacteria and found in animal foods; plants don't contain any. While some have claimed that vitamin K_2 is a separate vitamin with its own role in the body, no research supports this.

A study comparing blood-clotting rates (a measure of vitamin K activity) showed no difference between vegans and meat-eaters, which suggests that vegans are getting plenty of vitamin K.[10] And studies have shown that vitamin K_1 supplements are effective in older people for reducing bone fracture risk.

Since bacteria in the colon produces vitamin K_2, vegans are getting this form of the vitamin anyway. Finally, the Institute of Medicine has not established any specific recommendations for vitamin K_2. We can say with assurance that vitamin K_2 is not a separate nutrient, and vegans do not need it in their diet.

OTHER VITAMINS AND MINERALS

Over the years, there has been some discussion about riboflavin (vitamin B_2) in a vegan diet since the main source of this nutrient in American diets is milk. But while riboflavin is found in only small amounts in many plant foods, a varied diet of grains, legumes, and vegetables provides plenty. Soyfoods are a particularly good source of riboflavin. We don't have a great deal of information about vegan intake, but the few studies that have been done show that vegans meet the RDA for riboflavin. Choosing soy (or other plant) milks that are fortified with this nutrient can provide extra insurance, but we don't think that vegans need to worry about riboflavin. We've listed the riboflavin content of plant foods on page 77.

Both vegans and omnivores need to pay attention to the mineral potassium. Since legumes are a good source of this nutrient, vegans tend to have somewhat higher intakes than meat-eaters. But it's not easy for anyone to meet the recommended daily intake of potassium, which is 4,700 milligrams, without a bit of planning. Including plenty of vegetables in your diet is the easiest way to meet potassium needs, but it's important to choose those that are especially potassium-rich. Best sources are certain leafy greens (beet greens, spinach, and Swiss chard), cooked tomato products and tomato juice, orange juice, sea vegetables, bananas, and legumes. The table on page 78 shows the best sources of potassium for vegans.

The mineral selenium is the only other nutrient that may be an issue for some vegans. It depends on where you live—or where your food comes from—since the amount of selenium in plant foods is dependent on the amount in the soil where the foods are grown. Evidence suggests that vegans in the United States and Canada get enough selenium. In parts of northern Europe, the selenium content of the soil is fairly low, however, and vegans may need to supplement. The table on page 79 reflects selenium content of plant foods grown in the United States.

RIBOFLAVIN CONTENT OF PLANT FOODS

Recommended intake is 1.1 micrograms for women and 1.3 micrograms for men.

Food	Riboflavin Content (in milligrams)
Breads, cereals, grains	
Barley, whole, ½ cup	0.26
Bran flakes, ¾ cup	0.42
Corn flakes, 1 cup	0.74
Pasta, enriched, ½ cup	0.15
Pasta, whole wheat, ½ cup	0.03
Quinoa, ½ cup	0.1
White bread, 1 slice	0.9
Whole wheat bread, 1 slice	.06
Vegetables	
Asparagus	0.06
Beet greens	0.2
Collard greens	0.10
Mushrooms	0.23
Peas	0.08
Spinach	0.21
Sweet potatoes	0.08
Sea vegetables (½ cup cooked)	
Dulse	0.14
Kombu	0.018
Nori	0.47
Wakame	1.64
Fruit	
Banana, 1 medium	0.09
Legumes (½ cup cooked)	
Kidney beans	0.05
Soybeans	0.24
Split peas	0.06
Soyfoods	
Soymilk, 1 cup	0.5 (varies by brand)
Veggie "meats," 1 ounce	0.17 (varies by brand)
Miscellaneous	
Nutritional yeast, Vegetarian Support Formula, 1 tablespoon	4.8
Marmite yeast extract, ½ teaspoon	0.42

POTASSIUM CONTENT OF PLANT FOODS

Recommended intake is 4,700 milligrams.

Food	Amount of Potassium (in milligrams)
Legumes (½ cup cooked)	
Black-eyed peas	239
Chickpeas	239
Kidney beans	358
Lentils	365
Lima beans	478
Navy beans	354
Pinto beans	373
Soybeans	443
Split peas	355
Vegetables (½ cup cooked unless otherwise noted)	
Beet greens	654
Beets	259
Plantain	465
Potato	296
Spinach	419
Squash, acorn	322
Sweet potato	475
Swiss chard	480
Tomato juice, 1 cup	556
Tomato sauce, canned	405
V-8 Juice, reduced sodium, 1 cup	1000
Sea vegetables (½ cup cooked)	
Dulse	1023
Kombu	1708
Nori	371
Fruit	
Banana, 1 medium	422
Orange juice, 1 cup	443

SELENIUM CONTENT OF PLANT FOODS

Recommended intake is 55 micrograms.
These numbers are from USDA and may not apply outside of the United States.
People in other countries should check the selenium content of local supplies.

Food	Selenium Content (in micrograms)
Breads, cereals, grains	
Barley, pearled, ½ cup cooked	6.8
Bran flakes, 1 cup	4.1
Bread, whole wheat, 1 slice	7.2
Grape-Nuts, ½ cup	5.3
Oatmeal, ½ cup cooked	6.3
Pasta, whole-wheat, ½ cup cooked	18.1
Rice, brown, ½ cup cooked	9.6
Legumes and soyfoods (½ cup cooked)	
Chickpeas	3
Lima beans	4.2
Pinto beans	5.3
Soybeans	6.3
Tofu, firm	12.5
Nuts and seeds	
Brazil nuts, 2 tablespoons	319

MEETING NUTRIENT NEEDS: PUTTING IT ALL TOGETHER

It's good to know the different sources of individual nutrients and how to meet your needs for each one. But planning a healthy diet by tracking intake of individual nutrients can quickly become overwhelming and confusing. And it's not necessary for vegans or anyone else to do so. In the next chapter, we'll provide simple guidelines for planning menus that bring together the information we've talked about so far. It's the Vegan Food Guide—and it makes planning vegan diets a breeze.

Vegan Diets, Minerals, and Hair Loss

Every so often, we hear from women who believe that they have been losing hair since going vegetarian or vegan. While there are no studies of this issue in vegans, there is research on general nutrition factors and hair loss.

Reasons for hair loss vary among individuals, and they are not necessarily related to diet. About one-third of all younger (premenopausal) women experience some hair loss at one time or another (and the vast majority of these women are not vegan). And it is an unavoidable fact of life that hair thins as we age. Women going through menopause may notice a significant thinning of their hair.

Hair loss can be associated with certain medical conditions, including thyroid problems, so if you are convinced that you are losing hair at an unusual rate, it's important to see a physician. Sometimes a dermatologist can diagnose the problem.

Rapid weight loss can cause an increase in hair loss, and the hair growth should return to normal after the weight loss ceases. Women who become vegan sometimes initially lose weight quickly and this might account for the hair loss.

At one time, there was a widespread belief that zinc deficiency was a common cause of hair loss, but zinc supplementation has not been shown to help. Some studies have linked low iron status to hair loss in women, and it is possible that iron levels that are at the lower end of normal may not support optimal hair growth.

The essential amino acid L-lysine plays a part in the absorption of iron and zinc, and vegans who don't eat many legumes could find themselves falling short on lysine. Iron supplementation alone doesn't always increase iron stores. But in one study, iron supplementation plus a supplement of 1.5 to 2 grams per day of L-lysine increased iron stores and decreased hair loss by half.[7] Other supplements, like excessive intakes of vitamin E and folic acid, can adversely affect hair growth.

Finally, women who feel they are losing hair may choose to shampoo less frequently in the belief that this will preserve their hair. This hasn't been shown to prevent hair loss. In fact, since everyone loses some hair on a daily basis, if you shampoo less often, you'll see more hair in the tub each time you shampoo, which may convince you that you are losing more hair.

continues

Vegan Diets, Minerals, and Hair Loss
continued

If you believe you are losing more hair than usual, be sure to consider other factors first. If you've recently lost weight, gone through menopause, are shampooing less often, are dealing with increased stress, or have been taking supplements of vitamin E or folic acid, any of those might be the culprit. If you think diet might be the cause, you may want to have your iron levels measured.

CHAPTER 7

THE VEGAN FOOD GUIDE

Food guides have been a part of nutrition education in the United States for nearly one hundred years. They've come a long way too. The first one, published in 1916, had five food groups: fruits and vegetables; meat, fish, and milk; cereals; simple sweets; and butter and wholesome fats. It was produced by the United States Department of Agriculture (USDA), the same group that produces the food guide pyramid for Americans today.

While pressure from agriculture and the food industry shapes current food guides and keeps them friendly to animal foods, the trend has been toward a greater emphasis on plant foods. Even so, government food guides are not especially useful for vegetarians, and they are all but useless for vegans. Therefore we need to create our own.

The food guide in this chapter is not the final word on planning a healthy vegan diet. No single food guide represents the only way to meet nutrient needs. And you don't need to follow these guidelines with meticulous attention every day. You won't keel over and die if one day you have only four servings of grains!

This is meant to point you towards a diet that is based on a variety of whole grains, legumes, nuts, fruits, and vegetables. The guide doesn't include items like chocolate chip cookies, potato chips, and wine. But that doesn't mean you can't have them. They just don't fit into the food groups that should be at the center of your diet.

THE VEGAN FOOD GROUPS

To translate nutrition information into simple menu-planning guidelines, we've divided foods into the following groups:

Whole Grains and Starchy Vegetables

These foods are high in fiber, and provide protein, iron, zinc, and B vitamins. We've included starchy vegetables like potatoes and sweet potatoes because their calorie content and nutrient profiles are similar to those of grains. Although it's always a good idea to choose whole grains, products like fortified cereals can sometimes make important contributions to the diet, especially for children and some athletes.

Legumes and Soyfoods

These are the most protein-rich of all plant foods, and they are among the few good dietary sources of the essential amino acid lysine for vegans. We recommend at least three to four servings of these foods every day for adults. Generally, one serving provides around 7 to 8 grams of protein, but many of the soyfoods, such as tempeh, veggie meats, and some types of tofu, are quite a bit higher. These foods are also important sources of minerals like iron and sometimes zinc. If your diet is based on a variety of whole grains, vegetables, and nuts, then the three recommended servings from this group are plenty. If you like to spend some discretionary calories on desserts, added fats, or more servings of fruit (which are very low in protein), shooting for four servings of legumes per day will make it easier to meet protein and lysine needs.

If you are new to beans, keep an open mind about them. They are central to some of the world's best cuisine and can add great interest to your diet. Chapter 8 has tips for easy preparation and gas-free enjoyment of beans. We've also provided alternative ways to meet protein needs. See "For Those Who Don't Like Legumes" on page 90.

Soyfoods are a special category of legumes that includes any food made from soybeans, such as tofu, soymilk, tempeh, and veggie meats. You don't have to eat soyfoods, but they can be valuable in vegan diets. Not only are they nutritious, but they are convenient for replacing meat and dairy products in meals. They make it super-easy to plan vegetarian diets that are healthful, varied, and delicious. There is lots of controversy about soy these days, and we clear that up in Chapter 15.

Although this group includes soymilk, it doesn't include almond, hemp, oat, or rice milk since they are almost always low in protein.

Nuts and Seeds

Some vegans shy away from nuts and seeds because of their high fat content. But moderate nut consumption improves cholesterol levels and can even help with weight control (see Chapter 13 for more on this). These foods are concentrated in calories, though, so a serving is small—just two tablespoons of a nut or seed butter or whole seeds, or ¼ cup of nuts. We suggest consuming one to two servings of these foods every day. Choose nuts more often than seeds; they usually have a healthier fat profile and their health benefits are impressive. If you are allergic to nuts, add another serving from the legumes and soyfoods group to your meals.

Vegetables

Vegetables rule when it comes to nutrient-dense foods. They are among the best sources of vitamins C and A and contain thousands of plant chemicals that might improve health. All vegetables are good for you, but leafy greens like kale, collards, spinach, and turnip greens pack an especially powerful nutritional punch. They are rich in vitamins A, C, and K, potassium, iron, folate, sometimes calcium, and a host of plant chemicals that are linked to everything from reduced risk for heart disease to better eyesight with aging. Most people who grew up eating greens feel they can't live without them, and many newcomers to this food agree. If, however, you need a more gradual introduction to them, try mixing small amounts of greens into soups and stews.

If you are pressed for time, frozen vegetables are a good alternative to fresh. They are almost always comparable in nutrient content and, in fact, sometimes have even higher levels of nutrients.

Fruits

Fruits are good sources of vitamins C and A as well as certain minerals, and they provide plenty of phytochemicals. While fruit juices can be a valuable source of nutrients, they should be used in moderation. Try to consume most fruits in their fresh, raw state if possible.

Fats

Added fats aren't essential in healthy vegan menus, but small amounts of the right ones can fit in a well-balanced diet. We've specified around two servings for adults (note: a serving is just a teaspoon). It's okay to have more, and people with very high calorie needs may consume quite a bit more. You may want to read over the guidelines for choosing healthy fats in Chapter 5.

Where's the "Calcium Group?"

Most food guides aimed at vegetarians have a "milk" group, with soymilk included as an alternative. Food guides for vegans often have a "calcium-rich foods" group. But this doesn't make sense. Except for fats, *all* of the food groups contain calcium-rich foods, so why not take advantage of this?

That's what we've done in the guide on page 88. Our food guide encourages you to choose a variety of foods to meet calcium needs. Be sure that your choices from the food groups include at least six to eight servings of calcium-rich foods per day. (Or you can make up the difference with a calcium supplement.)

USING THE VEGAN FOOD GUIDE

The vegan food guide is aimed at helping adults meet *minimum* requirements for nutrients. (We'll provide guidelines for children in Chapter 10.) If you consume just what the guide specifies, it will provide you with approximately 1,600 calories. Since most adults need a higher calorie intake, you can meet your energy needs by boosting intakes from all of the food groups.

Again, make sure that you are including at least six to eight servings per day of calcium-rich foods. These are listed in the right-hand column of the food guide. For example, ½ cup of calcium-set tofu counts as a serving from the protein-rich foods group and also as one of your servings of a calcium-rich food. Or, if you include a cup of cooked kale with dinner, it counts as a serving of vegetables and also a serving of a calcium-rich food.

In a couple of cases, serving sizes need to be adjusted in order for a food to count as a calcium-rich choice. While a whole cup of soymilk is one serving from the protein-rich foods group, because it is so high in calcium, it counts as two servings of a calcium-rich food. And two navel oranges equal a single calcium-rich serving even though they cover two of your recommended fruit servings.

The food guide on page 88 includes some additional tips for making choices within each group.

It's easy to use the food guide to pull together vegan menus that are healthy and delicious. The three menus on pages 95 to 98 will give you several ideas for planning meals to meet different calorie levels.

In addition, the following supplements or fortified foods will ensure that you get adequate vitamin B_{12}, iodine, vitamin D, and omega-3 fats.

VEGAN FOOD GUIDE

Vegan Food Groups	Include at least 6 to 8 servings per day of these calcium-rich foods
Whole grains and starchy vegetables 5 or more servings per day A serving is ½ cup cooked cereal, pasta, rice, or other grain, 1 ounce ready-to-eat cereal, 1 slice bread, one 6-inch corn tortilla, ½ cup white or sweet potato or corn.	1 ounce calcium-fortified cereal
Refined grains like regular pasta fit into this group as well. It's a good idea to choose mostly whole grains.	
Legumes and soyfoods: 3 to 4 or more servings per day A serving is ½ cup cooked beans, tofu, tempeh, 1 ounce mock meat, 1 cup fortified soymilk, ¾ cup (6 ounces) fortified soy yogurt, 2 tablespoons peanut butter, ¼ cup peanuts, or ¼ cup soynuts.	½ cup tempeh, calcium-set tofu, or soybeans; ¼ cup soynuts; ¾ cup fortified yogurt; or 1 cup fortified soymilk (in this case, 1 serving of soymilk, which is 1 cup, equals 2 servings of a calcium-rich food).
See "For Those Who Don't Like Legumes" on page 90 for ideas on bean-free meal planning.	
Nuts and seeds 1 to 2 servings daily A serving is ¼ cup whole nuts, 2 tablespoons seeds, or 2 tablespoons nut or seed butter	¼ cup almonds or 2 tablespoons almond butter, tahini
Vegetables 5 servings or more A serving is ½ cup cooked vegetable, 1 cup raw vegetable, ½ cup vegetable juice	½ cup cooked or 1 cup raw bok choy, broccoli, collard greens, Chinese cabbage, kale, mustard greens, okra, ½ cup calcium-fortified tomato juice
Aim for a variety of leafy greens and bright yellow and orange vegetables.	
Fruits 2 or more servings per day A serving is 1 medium fresh fruit, ½ cup cooked or cut-up fruit, ½ cup fruit juice, ¼ cup dried fruit	½ cup calcium-fortified fruit juice, ¼ cup dried figs, 2 navel oranges
Include good sources of vitamin C, such as citrus fruits, cantaloupe, kiwifruit, papaya, and mangos with meals to increase absorption of iron.	
Fats 2 servings per day A serving is 1 teaspoon vegetable oil or soft margarine	

Vitamin B$_{12}$:
- Two servings per day of fortified foods providing 1.5 to 2.5 micrograms of vitamin B$_{12}$ per serving OR
- 25 to 100 micrograms per day from a chewable or sublingual supplement OR
- 1,000 micrograms twice per week from a chewable or sublingual supplement

Iodine:
- 75 to 150 micrograms three to four days per week (or ¼ teaspoon of iodized salt per day)

Vitamin D:
- 1,000 IU (25 micrograms) per day unless you are certain you are getting adequate sun exposure

Omega-3 Fats:
- DHA: A supplement providing 200 to 300 micrograms (of DHA or DHA plus EPA combined) from algae every two or three days (or every day for people over sixty)
- Alpha-linolenic acid: Be sure that your diet includes three to four servings per day from the following list.

1 teaspoon canola oil
¼ teaspoon flaxseed oil
⅔ teaspoon hempseed oil
1 teaspoon walnut oil
2 teaspoons ground English walnuts or 1 walnut half
1 teaspoon ground flaxseeds
½ cup cooked soybeans
1 cup firm tofu
1 cup tempeh
2 tablespoons soynuts

For Those Who Don't Like Legumes

If you're beginning a transition to a vegan diet you may not have much experience with beans. Most Americans rarely eat them. Soyfoods and other legumes make it especially easy to meet protein needs on a vegan diet, but they aren't absolutely essential to balanced meal planning. The real issue when you drop these foods from your diet is that it becomes more of a challenge to meet the needs for the essential amino acid lysine. If you choose not to eat legumes, you'll need to add three servings of other lysine-rich foods to your diet. A serving is one cup of quinoa, ¼ cup of pistachios, or ½ cup of cashews. This is in addition to the five servings of grains and one serving of nuts that are already recommended in the food guide.

Consider introducing beans to your meals gradually if they are new to your diet. Start out with one serving of legumes per day—maybe a hummus sandwich or bean burrito—plus one serving of a soyfood. Replace the third recommended serving with a lysine-rich food like ¼ cup of pistachios.

Because legumes are the most protein dense of all foods, diets require a bit more attention to planning when legume intake is limited. If you aren't consuming any legumes or soyfoods, make sure you are getting most of your calories from whole grains, vegetables, and nuts. Limit fruit and other low-protein foods like added fats, desserts, and alcohol.

WHOLE VERSUS PROCESSED FOODS: FINDING A BALANCE

It's easier than ever to plan healthy and interesting vegan meals because of the array of convenience products like veggie meats and cheeses and boxed and frozen dinners. Although many forms of processing strip away nutrients from foods or add undesirable ingredients, processed foods have a long and nutritionally important history in many world cuisines. Tofu and soymilk are two examples of processed foods that play a significant role in Asian cuisine.

While it is a good idea to build your diet around a variety of whole plant foods, moderate amounts of foods that don't carry the "whole foods" label can play a role, and sometimes an important one, in healthy vegan diets. For many, including veggie burgers, fortified plant milks, pasta sauce from a jar, instant soup, and other convenience foods makes vegan meal planning more realistic. It can improve the chances that you will meet nutrient needs and thrive on a vegan diet, and it can be especially important for children. Athletes and others with high calorie needs can also benefit from more processed foods.

Too often we have seen an unwavering commitment to eliminating all processed foods from meals morph into a restrictive eating pattern that is marginal in protein and fat and falls short of providing enough calories. Sadly, the result is that many people on this kind of regimen decide that a vegan diet is ruining their health or they find it unsatisfying and difficult, and they return to eating animal foods. On the other hand, we have rarely seen these kinds of problems in vegans who are more liberal in their food choices—enjoying veggie burgers, a drizzle of olive oil on salads, a sweet treat now and then, and whatever convenience products it takes to keep their vegan diet nutrient-rich and realistic.

The point isn't that you must eat processed foods to be healthy; it's that there is a reasonable way to balance healthy food choices with convenience if you wish to do so. A diet based on veggie meats and protein bars is not the best way to meet nutrient needs. But if a moderate use of processed foods makes it easy to stick with a vegan diet, then enjoying them will help you reap the health benefits of plant-based eating and support your commitment to a diet that reduces animal suffering.

ALLERGIES AND FOOD INTOLERANCES

Food allergies are an immune response to a protein that the body perceives as "foreign." The immune system reacts by producing antibodies, which can trigger skin rashes, nausea, or respiratory symptoms. Approximately 6 to 8 percent of children have food allergies and at least half outgrow them by adulthood. Food allergies affect only 2 to 4 percent of adults.

If you think you might be allergic to certain foods, it's a good idea to get tested by a qualified health professional and possibly get a second opinion from a professional who does a different type of testing. The number of people who believe they have allergies is much higher than the number who actually test positive for them. As an adult, you may no longer be allergic to foods that caused problems for you as a child.

Although any protein can cause allergies, eight foods account for more than 90 percent of food allergies. These are milk, eggs, fish, shellfish, tree nuts, peanuts, soy, and wheat. Of these, only tree nuts, peanuts, soy, and wheat are of concern to vegans. And peanut and tree nut allergies are the ones that are most likely to persist beyond childhood. Allergies to soy are relatively uncommon in both children and adults, and they are also unlikely to cause severe symptoms like respiratory problems. Wheat allergy is not the same as celiac disease, which is an intolerance to all sources of the protein gluten. People with wheat allergy need to avoid wheat but can usually consume other sources of gluten like barley. However, if you have a wheat allergy, the growing availability of gluten-free products makes it easier to plan a healthy diet.

There is no treatment for food allergies; if you have them, the only solution is to avoid all foods that cause reactions. Vegans who have multiple allergies face some challenges, but once you understand what you can and can't eat, and begin to explore alternatives, you may find that planning healthy and satisfying meals is easier than you think.

For people with the most common plant-food allergies—nuts, peanuts, soy, and wheat—there are plenty of foods to enjoy on the menu, such as quinoa, oats, rice, potatoes, millet, corn tortillas, certain types of Asian noodles, sunflower seeds, tahini, beans, vegetables, and fruits. Most people with allergies to tree nuts can safely eat coconuts.

People with allergies should carefully read labels, of course, since soy, wheat, and nuts can turn up where you might not expect to find them. Food labels include a list of common allergens at the end of the ingredient list.

Although it's easy to be vegan without shopping outside of conventional supermarkets, people with allergies may want to explore natural foods stores and Asian groceries as a way of expanding their choices.

Be sure to look at the online stores listed in the resource section of this book—they have great specialty items for people with allergies.

The following is one example of a vegan menu for someone with allergies to soy, tree nuts, peanuts, and wheat.

BREAKFAST

▸ Oatmeal with toasted sunflower seeds, chopped dried figs, and calcium-fortified rice milk

▸ Fresh fruit

SNACK

▸ Coconut milk yogurt

LUNCH

▸ Tostadas: corn tortillas topped with refried pinto beans, avocado, salsa, chopped raw vegetables, and Daiya cheese (a vegan cheese that is also free of soy)

▸ Fresh fruit

SNACK

▸ Rice crackers with sunflower seed butter

DINNER

▸ Rice noodles tossed with steamed vegetables and a sauce of tahini and lemon juice

▸ Salad with vinaigrette dressing

Food Intolerances

Food intolerances are different from allergies. Allergic reactions involve the immune system and are usually an all-or-nothing proposition. Even tiny amounts of the offending food can cause a problem. Food intolerances can be dose-related, meaning that the offending food can be consumed in small quantities. Intolerances are the result of different factors, such as decreased production of a particular enzyme, and they often cause digestive problems. The most common by far is lactose intolerance—a decreased ability to digest the sugar in milk. Fortunately, vegans don't have to worry about this.

New vegans who aren't used to eating legumes and high-fiber foods may experience another type of intolerance that results from increased gas production and intestinal discomfort.

It's hard to convince people that gas is good for them, but it may very well be true! The sugars in beans can't be digested by human enzymes, so they travel intact to the colon, where friendly bacteria reside. These bacteria break down the sugars, producing gas in the process. Eating more of these sugars in beans actually promotes the growth of these bacteria, and that's a good thing, since they contribute to an environment in the colon that lowers the risk for cancer.

Healthy or not, gas can be uncomfortable, not to mention embarrassing. Over time, however, you're likely to find that you adjust to bean consumption and feel much less gas-y. Exercise, such as a walk after dinner, may help. In the meantime, there are two options:

Emphasize less gas-y beans in your diet. Lentils and split peas tend to produce less gas.

Rinse beans several times during soaking. First, place beans and soaking water in a large pot and bring the water to a boil. Boil for two minutes. Drain the beans and add fresh water. Soak the beans in the refrigerator for six hours. Drain and add fresh water for cooking.

1,600 CALORIE MENU

	Grains and starchy vegetables	Legumes and soyfoods	Nuts and seeds	Vegetables	Fruit	Fats	Calcium-rich foods
Breakfast							
½ cup oatmeal	1						
1 cup fortified soymilk		1					2
½ cup calcium-fortified orange juice					1		1
1 slice whole wheat toast	1						
1 tablespoon jam							
Lunch							
1 cup tomato-lentil soup		1		1			
6 whole-grain crackers	1						
½ cup carrot juice				1			
Green salad with vinaigrette dressing with 1 teaspoon olive oil				1		1	
Snack							
Apple slices with 2 tablespoons almond butter			1		1		1
Dinner							
Veggie burger		1					
Small baked sweet potato	1						
2 cups sautéed broccoli and cauliflower sautéed in 1 teaspoon olive oil				4		1	2
Snack							
1 cup bran flakes	1						
1 cup soymilk		1					2
Total Food Group Servings	5	4	1	7	2	2	8

2,000 CALORIE MENU

	Grains and starchy vegetables	Legumes and soyfoods	Nuts and seeds	Vegetables	Fruit	Fats	Calcium-rich foods
Breakfast							
1 cup tofu and ¼ cup mushrooms scrambled in 1 teaspoon margarine		2		½		1	2
1 slice whole-wheat toast	1						
2 tablespoons almond butter			1				1
1 cup strawberries					1		
Snack							
Oatmeal cookie	1						
Lunch							
Hummus sandwiches made from 3 following items:							
2 four-inch whole wheat pita pockets	2						
½ cup hummus		1					1
Chopped tomatoes and lettuce				1			
1 cup melon cubes					1		
Snack							
¼ cup mixed nuts			1				
½ cup grapes					1		
Dinner							
1 cup baked beans topped with 2 tablespoons shredded vegan cheese		2					
1 cup quinoa and corn mixed	2						
2 cups steamed collard greens sautéed in 1 teaspoon olive oil				4		1	4
Salad with squeeze of lemon, herbs, and 1 teaspoon olive oil				1		1	
Total Food Group Servings	6	5	2	6½	3	3	8

2,500 CALORIE MENU

	Grains and starchy vegetables	Legumes and soyfoods	Nuts and seeds	Vegetables	Fruit	Fats	Calcium-rich foods
Breakfast							
1 cup muesli topped with 1 teaspoon ground flaxseed	2		½				
1 cup fortified soymilk		1					2
1 slice whole-wheat toast	1						
2 tablespoons peanut butter		1					
Banana					1		
Lunch							
Tempeh Reuben made from 4 following items:							
2 slices rye bread	2						
3 ounces marinated tempeh strips		1					
1 slice vegan cheese							1
¼ cup sauerkraut				½			
1 ounce baked tortilla chips	1						
½ cup carrot juice				1			
1 cup melon cubes					1		
Snack							
¾ cup vegan lemon yogurt		1					1
½ cup blueberries					1		

continues

2,500 CALORIE MENU

continued

	Grains and starchy vegetables	Legumes and soyfoods	Nuts and seeds	Vegetables	Fruit	Fats	Calcium-rich foods
Dinner							
Pasta with fresh vegetables and pine nuts made from 5 following items:							
1 cup pasta	2						
2 cups steamed broccoli, carrots, and snow peas				4			2
1 cup cannellini beans		2					
2 teaspoons olive oil						2	
2 tablespoons toasted pine nuts			1				
½ cup fresh fruit salad					1		
Green salad with vinaigrette using 1 teaspoon olive oil				1		1	
Snack							
1 brownie							
Total Food Group Servings	8	6	1½	6½	4	3	6

Stocking the Vegan Pantry

Your vegan pantry will depend on your food preferences, of course, as well as your cooking style. Gourmet cooks may have shelves filled with specialty condiments and exotic ingredients from international grocery stores, while non-cooks may opt for a little (or a lot) more convenience.

You can find the majority of these foods in any conventional grocery store. A few require a trip to a natural foods store, and depending on where you live, some may be available only by mail order.

Pantry Basics

Dried and canned beans: You'll find black, navy, garbanzo, kidney, pinto, and lima beans, plus lentils, black-eyed peas, and split peas in most grocery stores. Check specialty stores for some other interesting options, including red adzuki beans, maroon and white speckled Anasazi beans, and mung beans (great for sprouting).

Grains: Because grains have a long shelf life, you can keep lots of them on hand. Each has its own unique taste and texture, and they are a great way to add interest to meals. Here are a few choices:

- **Barley:** One of the oldest cultivated foods in the world, this has a chewy quality and mild taste. Pearled barley has the outer bran removed and cooks more quickly but is still high in fiber.
- **Bulgur:** A fast-food type of grain, this is whole wheat that has been precooked and then dried. It's common in Middle Eastern cooking, where it's used to make tabouli.
- **Couscous:** Common in the cooking of North Africa, this is made from steamed, dried wheat and it cooks very quickly.
- **Millet:** Americans think of this as bird seed, but it's widely used in African and Asian cuisines.
- **Quinoa:** This high-protein grain was a staple in the diet of the Incas, who called it the "mother grain." Quinoa is fast-cooking and high in protein, which has made it very popular among modern cooks. It has a natural soap-like coating to protect it from pests, so be sure to rinse it thoroughly before cooking.

continues

Stocking the Vegan Pantry
continued

- **Wheat berries:** A slow-cooking grain with a very chewy quality, it's usually mixed with other grains.

Italian pasta: This type of pasta comes in a host of wonderful shapes, and many are available in whole-wheat versions.

Asian pasta: Modern choices include mung bean noodles, soba noodles (Japanese buckwheat noodles), ramen, and udon.

Rolled or steel-cut oats and other hot cereals

Breads and whole-grain crackers

Whole-wheat and corn tortillas

Nuts: This list includes almonds, cashews, hazelnuts, peanuts, walnuts, pecans, and pine nuts. Peanuts are an honorary member of this group since they are actually legumes. So are soynuts, which are soybeans that have been soaked and roasted until they are crunchy.

Seeds: Sesame, sunflower, and pumpkin seeds

Vegetable oils: Extra-virgin olive oil and canola oil are basics that will cover most of your oil needs. See Chapter 5 for an extensive discussion of oils.

Canned tomato products: Prepared pasta sauce, tomato paste, whole and diced tomatoes, crushed tomatoes, and tomato sauce are all handy for making soups, stews, and other dishes.

Vegetable broth: If you don't have time to make homemade vegetable stock, vegetable broth or bouillon cubes or powder are available.

Textured vegetable protein (TVP™): A dry soy-protein product; rehydrate with boiling water and add to spaghetti sauce for a ground beef substitute.

Sea vegetables: Look for dulse, arame, nori, hijiki, kombu, laver, and others. Most are available in dried form and are a quick addition to soups. Nori is used to make the wraps for sushi.

Coconut milk: Look for reduced-fat coconut milk in the international foods section of the grocery store. It's an essential addition to many Thai and Indian dishes.

continues

Stocking the Vegan Pantry
continued

Refrigerator Basics

This list includes items that must always be refrigerated as well as those that should be refrigerated after they have been opened.

Nut butters: Peanut and almond butters are staples. There are plenty of other choices, too, although they tend to be pricey. Nut butters are good for sandwiches or to spread on apple slices, but they also can be thinned with water and seasoned to make great sauces for grains and vegetables.

Sesame tahini: An essential ingredient in homemade hummus that is equally good for sauces and dressings.

Miso: Absolutely essential in Japanese cooking, it is also considered a staple by most vegans.

Fortified plant milks: Soymilk is the most nutritious and protein-rich, but you might also enjoy almond, oat, hempseed, and rice milk.

Fresh or aseptically packaged tofu: Choose firm tofu for scrambles and stir-fries, soft or silken for sauces and soups.

Tempeh: An ancient food from Indonesia, this cake of fermented soybeans has an indescribably delicious flavor. It's a great protein source to toss into stir-fried dishes. You can read more about tempeh and other soy products in Chapter 8.

Vital wheat gluten: A flour made from wheat protein, it's used to create seitan, which has a chewy, meat-like texture. You can also buy prepared seitan.

Dried fruits: Figs, apricots, prunes, and raisins.

Vegan mayonnaise: There are several brands on the market, but Vegenaise, made by the Follow Your Heart Company, is the most popular choice.

Vegan margarine: Most vegan cooks swear by the Earth Balance brand, which is widely available and does not contain hydrogenated oils.

Veggie meats: Look for these in the frozen and refrigerated section of grocery stores. Be sure to check labels since some contain dairy and eggs.

continues

Stocking the Vegan Pantry
continued

Vegan cheeses, cream cheese, sour cream and yogurt: These are made from soy, almonds, hempseed, and even coconut.

Fruits and vegetables

Lemons and limes

White and sweet potatoes

Onions and fresh garlic

Condiments: Ketchup, mustard, relish, pickles, salsa, barbecue sauce, black and green olives—the same condiments that you'll find in the refrigerators of most omnivores, vegetarians, and vegans alike.

Freezer Basics

Frozen corn and peas: Nice to have on hand to toss into grain salads. They do not need to be cooked.

Premade pizza shells

Vegan ice cream

Backup: The freezer is a good place to store extra packages of tempeh, seitan, and veggie meats, as well as nuts and seeds (which can turn rancid in the cupboard and even in the refrigerator after a long enough time).

Basic Condiments

Iodized salt: Many vegan cookbooks suggest using sea salt. But sea salt has the same effects on blood pressure and calcium loss as any other salt—and it's not a reliable source of iodine. So use salt sparingly, and when you do, choose plain iodized salt.

Vegan Worcestershire sauce: Traditionally, this sauce is made with fish (anchovies), but low-sodium Worcestershire sauce is often vegan. Or look for one that says "vegetarian" on the label.

Jams, jellies, and preserves

Tamari: A more authentic version of soy sauce.

continues

Stocking the Vegan Pantry
continued

Nutritional yeast: Look for Red Star brand Vegetarian Support Formula because that's the type that provides vitamin B$_{12}$.

Vinegars: Apple cider, balsamic, and white wine vinegar will cover most of your needs, but there are many others available. Rice vinegar is great for adding an authentic Asian flavor to stir-fried dishes.

More Luxurious Condiments

Cooking enthusiasts will want to have these on hand, but even if you don't consider yourself a "gourmet" chef, they can add fast, easy flavor to basic grain, bean, and tofu dishes.

- Chili paste
- Hoisin sauce
- Teriyaki sauce
- Chutney
- Curry paste
- Artichoke hearts
- Sundried tomatoes packed in oil
- Roasted red bell peppers
- Olive tapenade
- Capers
- Liquid smoke
- Mirin
- Dried shiitake mushrooms

Baking

Ground flaxseed or EnerG egg replacer or soy flour: These are used for replacing eggs.

Agar powders or flakes: Boil this seaweed in water or juice to produce a gelatin-like product. You'll find it in natural foods stores or Asian markets.

Baking powder, baking soda, flours

Chickpea flour: Natural foods and specialty stores are packed with all kinds of flours. Chickpea flour is a "basic" because when it is used to thicken vegetable broth, it makes a wonderful gravy to pour over mashed potatoes and vegan Thanksgiving stuffing. In Indian groceries, it's usually called *besan*.

Unsweetened cocoa powder

continues

Stocking the Vegan Pantry
continued

Sweeteners: There are plenty of great vegan sweeteners on the market, including

beet sugar, rice syrup, barley malt syrup, and maple syrup.

Blackstrap molasses: Add small amounts to stews and bean dishes; its bold, rugged flavor means that a little goes a long way. Blackstrap molasses (*not* regular molasses) is a good source of iron and calcium.

Vanilla and lemon extracts

Bread crumbs

Wheat germ

Herbs and Spices

The sky's the limit when it comes to herbs and spices, especially if you love to cook and experiment with ethnic dishes. If you want just the basics, here's what to keep on hand:

- Allspice
- Basil
- Bay leaves
- Cayenne powder
- Chili powder
- Cinnamon
- Coriander
- Cumin
- Curry powder
- Garlic powder
- Ginger
- Nutmeg
- Onion powder
- Oregano
- Paprika
- Parsley
- Rosemary
- Savory
- Thyme
- Turmeric

Beverages

Coffee, tea, wine, beer, soft drinks, juices, and whatever else is popular in your home.

CHAPTER 8

MAKING THE TRANSITION TO A VEGAN DIET

When you go meatless and dairy-free, what on earth do you eat? Some of the best food you've ever tasted!

It would seem that dropping entire food categories from your menus would leave a diet that feels very restricted. But upon going vegan, many people find that their food horizons actually expand as they explore new menu items like crusty barbecued Indonesian tempeh, sweet almond milk, crispy falafel croquettes, and tangy sesame butter sauce. Dining at a vegan table is anything but dull!

But what if exotic fare isn't your thing? What if you have neither the patience nor time to follow a recipe? That's fine. You can build healthful and appealing vegan meals around convenience foods and easily prepared dishes—old standbys that have been a part of your diet all of your life, like spaghetti with marinara sauce.

There are plenty of wonderful cookbooks and recipe websites for vegans, and we've listed several in the resource section. But you can be a happy, healthy vegan without ever cracking open a cookbook. After all, it doesn't take much instruction to bake a potato, flavor beans with onions and salsa, and round out the meal with steamed spinach. Much of the cooking that people do—whether or not they are vegan—is just this type of casual, unstructured preparation.

GETTING STARTED

It's not hard to create great vegan meals and find substitutes for the foods you've always enjoyed. Yes, there is a learning curve as you switch from the diet you've always known to one that is based on plant foods. But if you take it one step at a time, going vegan is a fun adventure.

Some people dive into a vegan diet and lifestyle overnight while others need to test the waters and make a gradual transition. The transition can occur in any number of ways, and it's up to you to decide what feels logical and practical. Don't assume that you have to go vegetarian—omitting meat while still eating eggs and dairy—as the first step toward veganism. Some people do, and that's fine, but it's not the only, or necessarily best, way to begin reducing your intake of animal products.

The tips in this chapter cover a broad range of big and small changes and offer options for different cooking and eating styles. Choose the ones that seem most realistic to begin with and then keep making changes at the pace that feels right for you.

Make Small, Easy Substitutions Right Away

These are the changes that don't require any real knowledge about cooking or meal planning. They won't make much difference in your meal preparation, but they will reduce your intake of animal foods immediately. For example, trade in cow's milk for plant-based milk, and start using vegan salad dressings, sour cream, and mayonnaise. Even if you are still unsure about going vegan, it's worth reducing animal food intake with these very easy changes.

Condiments are a good way to make simple substitutions that build fast flavor into foods. Some all-American favorites like mustard, relish, and ketchup are already vegan. For those products that typically contain animal ingredients, here are some winning substitutes.

- Look for creamy vegan salad dressings in the store, or just go with an easy and healthy option—olive oil and vinegar.

- Try Vegenaise brand vegan mayonnaise; believe it or not, it's better than regular commercial mayonnaise.
- Choose low-sodium Worcestershire sauce, which is usually free of anchovies.
- Trade vegetable broth or bouillon for chicken broth in recipes.
- Serve mushroom gravy on potatoes instead of meat-based gravy.

If you are accustomed to using cow's milk as a beverage, with cereal, or in cooking and baking, look into some of the alternatives. Try milks made from soy, rice, hemp, oats, or almonds on cereal, in baking, to make chocolate pudding, or to wash down a cookie. Look for choices that are fortified with calcium and vitamin D. If you don't like one, try another. It may take a few attempts, but with the vast array of products, you'll find something that suits you.

Most cheese alternatives contain small amounts of the milk protein casein, but there are some wonderful, completely vegan choices. The Follow Your Heart Company, a leader in the production of delicious vegan foods, makes Vegan Gourmet cheese in a variety of flavors. We also love Daiya and Teese, which are great to melt over pasta or on a pizza. For a vegan wine and cheese party, try Sheese, which is made in Scotland and crafted in a variety of styles, including Gouda, Edam and smoked Cheddar. You don't need to make the substitutions all at once; one week, try a nondairy milk, then the next, try a nondairy cheese. Check the resources section at the end of this book for where to order these products if your local natural foods store doesn't carry them.

Here are additional ideas for phasing dairy out of your meals:

- Spread your morning bagel with nondairy cream cheese made by either Tofutti or Follow Your Heart. Most larger grocery stores carry one of these brands in the natural foods section.
- Spoon a few dollops of vegan sour cream into soup or on top of burritos. Again, we recommend Tofutti and Follow Your Heart for these products.

- Try Mocha Mix or other nondairy creamers in coffee. Or make a soymilk foam for cappuccino.
- Have fun exploring the vast array of nondairy frozen desserts. Who needs ice cream when there is Coconut Bliss in the world?
- Everything that replaces dairy in your diet doesn't have to be an analogue. Spread almond butter or mashed avocado on toast instead of butter for a more healthful choice and a nice change of pace. Or flavor tofu with salt and herbs and crumble it on top of a vegan pizza.
- Try to think a little further outside the box. We love this recipe from *The Ultimate Uncheese Cookbook* by Joanne Stepaniak. It tastes like old-fashioned Cheez Whiz. Blend together one 15-ounce can of drained, rinsed Great northern beans, ½ cup roasted red peppers or pimento pieces, 6 to 8 tablespoons nutritional yeast flakes, 3 tablespoons fresh lemon juice, 2 to 3 tablespoons tahini, ½ teaspoon prepared yellow mustard, ½ teaspoon salt, and ¼ teaspoon each of garlic and onion powder.

Identify Ten Great Vegan Dinner Menus

Start with what you know. What's on family menus that is already vegan or could be vegan with just a tweak or two? How about pasta with marinara sauce? Or tomato soup? (Prepare it with soymilk instead of cow's milk.) Make Sloppy Joes using a canned sauce and meatless "ground beef." Peanut butter and jelly sandwiches are vegan and so is hummus. Starting with foods that are familiar can be a good way to help children make a smooth transition to plant-based meals.

Next, spend some time with cookbooks, the Internet, and your own recipe collection to identify seven to ten easy vegan dinners that you like and can prepare without much fuss (unless you like to fuss, of course). That's as much variety as most omnivores enjoy, and families are usually very happy with a ten-day cycle of their favorite meals. Over time, you'll probably grow tired of some and replace them with others, but for starters, this short list of meals will get you through your first months as a vegan.

Where's the Meat?

When you want something "meaty," the selection of vegan choices these days is amazing. Check the frozen and refrigerated sections of natural foods stores as well as your regular grocery store. You'll find vegan burgers, sausages, hotdogs, sandwich slices, pepperoni, Canadian bacon, pulled pork, chicken nuggets, ground beef, and much more. Different options appeal to different palates, so keep tasting until you find the items that you and your family enjoy. Look for products made by Gardein, Field Roast, Tofurky, Lightlife, and Yves, among others.

This is a chance to quickly eliminate some of the most harmful foods in omnivore diets. For example, cured and processed meats are especially unhealthy foods. Try a vegan substitute like Tofurky lunch meats, which taste very similar to their meat-derived counterparts.

And vegans can look to Asian cuisine for tofu and tempeh, two of the best meat substitutes. Read more about these staples of Asian diets in the Soyfoods Primer on pages 119–123. Both can be cubed, marinated in a simple sauce (try any barbecue, Thai peanut, or Teriyaki sauce), and then baked or sautéed. Serve them over rice or tossed with cooked vegetables.

In many (healthier) cultures, meat is used sparingly to flavor food, not as the focus of the meal. Vegans should plan meals in a similar fashion. Serve a platter of brown rice tossed with ¼ cup of almonds and topped with teriyaki-flavored sautéed veggies. Or make pasta the center of your plate, tossed with some garbanzo beans, vegan Parmesan cheese, and a big serving of steamed vegetables.

Take Advantage of Convenience Foods

You don't have to be a sophisticated or creative cook in order to follow a vegan diet. It's nice to know a few basics—how to bake a potato, cook brown rice, and steam vegetables—but that's no more or less than any-one, eating any type of diet, needs to know.

Anyone can make these ten vegan dinners:

- Baked potato topped with vegan baked beans and shredded soy cheese and accompanied by frozen spinach sautéed in olive oil.
- Veggie burger on a roll with salad and prepared salad dressing.
- Pasta salad: Toss cooked pasta with canned chick peas, onions, chopped raw vegetables, and vegan mayonnaise.
- Burritos: Use leftover beans or canned vegan refried beans. Spoon onto warm tortillas, roll them up, and top with chopped tomatoes and cubes of avocado.
- Pasta with sauce from a jar (add sautéed veggies or soy sausage for your own "homemade" touch).
- Chili beans with veggie burger crumbles served over rice with steamed carrots.
- Soup and salad. Progresso makes vegan lentil soup. Campbell's Tomato Soup—very possibly the most famous soup in America—is vegan. Just add plain soymilk. Make it go a little farther with a healthful addition like pasta, rice, or beans. Trader Joe's and Imagine Foods both make good vegan soups in aseptic boxes.
- Taco salad: Toss together greens, chopped tomato, chopped onion, rinsed canned black beans, defrosted corn, and cubes of avocado. Dress with olive oil and lime or lemon juice and top with a handful of crushed tortilla chips.
- Chunks of firm tofu and frozen vegetables marinated in peanut or teriyaki sauce (find both in the ethnic foods section of the gro-cery store). Sauté in a little bit of canola oil and serve over rice or noodles.
- Whole-grain main-dish salad: This is a great way to use up left-over cooked grains. Toss brown rice, couscous, barley, or what-ever you have on hand with chopped onion, defrosted frozen peas and corn, sunflower seeds, and rinsed canned beans. Top with your favorite dressing or with olive oil and lemon juice.

Look to Ethnic Cuisine

Some of the best eating patterns in the world—from both a culinary and health standpoint—are based on plant foods. When you start exploring meals from Italy, India, Mexico, China, Thailand, and other exotic locales, it will open up your world to the best of vegan cuisine. Look in cookbooks and online for recipes for pasta or Asian noodle dishes, curries, stir-fries, and pilafs (made with grains, nuts, and dried fruits). And look for ethnic restaurants when eating out since they are likely to have a good choice of vegan dishes.

Experiment with Beans

Most Americans didn't grow up eating beans, which is too bad. Legumes are super nutritious foods and among the world's cheapest and most abundant sources of protein. That's why beans have played a role in the diets of nearly every culture. If you can't get organized enough to cook beans from scratch, it's fine to use canned. Try bean dishes that are familiar, like baked beans (you can buy the canned vegan variety), bean burritos, and lentil and split pea soups.

One way to update your attitude about this group of foods is to become familiar with their use in other cultures. Chickpeas simmered in fresh tomato sauce, along with pasta and a glass of Chianti is a meal featuring the traditional flavors of Sicily. Other wonderful bean-based delicacies: garlic-infused Cuban black beans, spicy Indian lentil curry, and lemony chickpea hummus from the Middle East. Truly, beans are anything but boring!

What to Do with Beans

It's a simple matter to turn cooked beans into a tasty dish. Here are some super-fast ideas for ways to flavor beans. Most of these dishes can be served over rice or other grains—or spooned over a baked potato.

Black, pinto, and kidney beans

- **Mexican-style beans:** For each cup of cooked beans, stir in ¼ cup salsa and ¼ cup corn kernels. Heat and serve over rice topped with shredded soy cheese or chopped avocado and tomatoes.
- **Mediterranean beans:** Sauté ½ cup chopped onion and 2 stalks celery in 3 tablespoons olive oil until tender. Stir in 2 cans beans (rinsed) or 3 cups cooked beans, 4 ounces sliced pimiento-stuffed green olives, and a 4-ounce can chopped chili peppers.

White beans (great northern, baby lima, or cannellini)

- **Beans with mushrooms:** Sauté 1½ cups sliced mushrooms in 2 tablespoons olive oil. Add 3 cups cooked beans and season with black pepper and fresh lemon juice. You might also add canned or chopped tomatoes.
- **Barbecued beans:** Mix 3 tablespoons prepared barbecue sauce into each cup of cooked beans.
- **Zesty beans with tomato sauce:** Mix 3 tablespoons prepared spaghetti sauce (try a spicy one) into each cup of cooked beans.
- **Italian-style beans with figs:** Sauté ¼ cup chopped onion and a clove of minced garlic in 1 tablespoon olive oil. Add 3 cups cooked beans and ½ cup chopped dried figs. Season with 1 teaspoon each dried basil and rosemary.
- **Hoppin' John:** Sauté 1 cup chopped onion and 2 minced garlic cloves in 3 tablespoons olive oil. Add 4 cups of beans and ¼ teaspoon ground cayenne pepper (more if you like your food very spicy). Add ¼ cup chopped veggie bacon (or a sprinkle of bacon bits) if you like. Prepare this dish with black-eyed peas for a traditional southern New Year's Day supper. It's supposed to bring good luck for the coming year.
- **Beans with apples and sausage:** Sauté ½ cup chopped onions in 2 tablespoons olive oil. Add 3 cups cooked beans, 1 diced apple, and 4 ounces vegan sausage (defrosted and crumbled). Simmer until everything is heated through and apples are tender.

All bean types

- **Sloppy Joes:** Add a 15-ounce can of Sloppy Joe sauce to two cups cooked beans. Heat and serve over whole-wheat hamburger rolls.
- **Bean and potato soup:** Sauté one cup chopped onions and 2 cloves minced garlic in 2 tablespoons olive oil. Add 2 cups diced potatoes, 2 cups cooked beans, and 8 cups vegetable broth. Simmer for 20 minutes until potatoes are tender. Season with basil and oregano.
- **Bean and grain salad:** Toss 3 cups of any cooked grain with 1 cup cooked beans. Season with bottled or homemade salad dressing. Add ¼ cup each of minced onion, chopped celery, and/or shredded carrots for added flavor and crunch.

Take Advantage of Familiar Favorites for Breakfast

Many people eat the same breakfast every single day, perhaps with a slight variation on the weekends. Hot or cold cereal with nondairy milk, toast with nut butter, juice, and fruit make a very hearty and healthy vegan breakfast that will suit the needs of most family members. Pancakes, vegan French toast, or scrambled tofu are good choices for more leisurely weekend breakfasts. Don't be afraid to think beyond traditional breakfast foods. A veggie burger or soup is just as good for breakfast as for dinner.

Identify Snacks, Treats, and Desserts that are Vegan

You might want to experiment with egg-free baking (see page 114) or look for baked goods and frozen desserts in the natural foods store. Old-fashioned, all-purpose cookbooks have recipes for fruit crumbles and crisps that are vegan—or that can be "veganized" by replacing butter with margarine. If you love all-American cuisine, take a look at the Betty Crocker Project (www.meettheshannons.net/p/betty-crocker -project.html), which aims to veganize every recipe in the *Betty Crocker Picture Cookbook* published in the 1950s.

Many snack chips are vegan and so are several brands of commercial cookies, including Oreos. Take a peek in the freezer section of your natural foods store, too, for frozen desserts such as Coconut Bliss, hempseed-based Tempt, and So Delicious products.

Learn to Bake without Eggs

The egg's main claim to fame is its role as a functional participant in cooking. In baking, it helps with leavening, and in savory foods, like veggie burgers, it's a binding agent. But other ingredients have those same properties, and there are plenty of effective ways to replace eggs in cooking.

To keep vegan loaves, burgers and croquettes from falling apart, add a little bit of flour, bread crumbs, or rolled oats.

For egg-free baking, you are likely to get better results by using refined flours since they are lighter and more easily leavened. (It's fine to use whole grains, though, just as long as you know to expect a somewhat heavier product.)

Look for recipes that call for just one or two eggs since it is easy to replicate them with a vegan version. Most cake mixes lend themselves well to vegan baking. For foods that don't require a great deal of leavening, like pancakes, you can simply eliminate the eggs and add an extra two tablespoons of water or soymilk.

Natural foods groceries carry commercial products like EnerG Egg Replacer and Bob's Red Mill Egg Replacer or try one of the following to replace eggs in baked goods.

For each egg:

- Grind 1 heaping tablespoon of whole flaxseed in a blender until it becomes a fine meal. Add 3 tablespoons cold water and blend until thick and viscous. The consistency is just like raw egg.
- Beat together 2 tablespoons water, 1 tablespoon oil, and 2 teaspoons baking powder.

- Whip 1 tablespoon plain agar powder (a seaweed product found in most natural foods stores) with 1 tablespoon water. Chill and then whip again.
- Mix 1 tablespoon full-fat soy flour with 3 tablespoons water.
- Mix together 1 tablespoon white vinegar and 1 teaspoon baking soda to make an instant, light foam.

Go Egg-Free for Breakfast and Lunch

When it comes to replacing eggs on the menu, there is nothing like tofu. Mash tofu and sauté it in vegan margarine with mushrooms and a sprinkle of nutritional yeast for "scrambled tofu." Or chop firm tofu and mix with onion, celery, and vegan mayonnaise for vegan egg salad. You may want to track down some black salt (called *kala namak*), which can be found in Indian groceries or ordered online. It smells and tastes exactly like egg yolks. Try it in scrambled tofu or in recipes for vegan omelets.

Pack Up Vegan Food to Go

There are thousands and thousands of vegan recipes for dinner and at-home meals. But you can brown-bag it vegan-style too. If your workplace has a microwave oven, you can enjoy instant soups packaged as individual servings (the kind in cardboard cups) or prepared burritos. If you don't have access to a microwave, take leftover beans, soups, or stews to work in a good quality thermos. Use the weekend to prepare a big pot of soup or beans and then freeze individual portions for grab-and-go meals to heat at work.

Or make sandwiches from vegan luncheon meats or hummus. Hummus-to-Go made by Wild Garden is a good choice when you don't have refrigeration since it comes in sealed individual-serving-size packages. Trail mix, instant oatmeal, and apples with almond butter are other tasty on-the-go snacks.

A great option for brown-bag lunches is a wrap sandwich that uses leftovers from dinner. Keep a stack of large whole-wheat flour tortillas in the refrigerator and try some of the combinations below for wrap fillings:

- Diced potatoes, chopped celery, capers, and sun-dried tomatoes. Add a dressing of hummus, lemon tahini, or vegan mayonnaise with Dijon mustard.
- Black or pinto beans with shredded Monterey Jack–style jalapeño soy cheese and chopped tomatoes.
- Shredded carrots, peanuts, and raisins mixed with vegan mayonnaise.
- Veggie burger crumbles tossed with sunflower seeds, shredded carrots, and tahini.
- Peanut butter and jelly. (Who says you can't have a PB&J wrap?)
- Rice, lentils, and shredded cabbage with sesame shiitake vinaigrette.
- Chopped chickpeas, onions, and celery mixed with vegan mayo and a dash of lemon juice.
- Baked tofu with spicy peanut sauce.
- Chopped tomatoes, carrots, and cucumber mixed into hummus.

Keep Learning

The variety of vegan products is growing like wildfire, and you'd be surprised by how many old-time favorites in the grocery store are vegan. As you explore, experiment, and taste, your menus will evolve, and you'll find solutions to menu-planning problems. Even longtime vegans find that their menus and diets develop over time based on new products and changing lives. Maybe you need to identify a list of restaurants where you can meet friends or take business clients or host a child's birthday party. If you entertain, you may need to gather ideas for a vegan cocktail party or for family get-togethers. The Internet is a valuable resource for these more specific issues.

VEGAN ON A BUDGET

Making the change to a vegan diet won't automatically save you money, but it's easy enough to plan healthy and enjoyable meals with a budget in mind. There's a balance, though: The best way to cut back on food expenses is to eat out less frequently and limit pricey convenience foods. But that usually translates to more time spent cooking, and not everyone has that time. Here are a few ideas that will help you save money without spending hours in the kitchen.

- Cook beans and grains from scratch but in large enough quantities to stretch for several meals. Leftovers don't have to be the same old thing. Serve black beans over rice the first night and then mixed with corn and salsa and wrapped in a corn tortilla the next. If you still have beans leftover, you can stretch them with a can of tomatoes for a third dinner. Or cook up a pot of chickpeas and use half to make hummus for sandwiches and half in a pasta and bean soup. The versatility of beans means that they can appear in meals throughout the week without getting boring.
- Get the most from higher-cost ingredients. Nuts, in particular, tend to be expensive, but a small amount goes a long way. One tablespoon of ground nuts mixed into a serving of cooked grains can add substantial flavor for very little cost. The same is true of more deluxe foods like sun-dried tomatoes, olives, and curry paste.
- No amount of leftovers is too small to save. If you have just a quarter cup of rice left, toss in some shredded carrots and a little bit of tahini and roll it up in a whole-wheat tortilla for a wrap sandwich. Little odds and ends in the refrigerator can often be pulled together into a salad or soup.
- Keep frozen vegetables on hand. They are just as nutritious as and often cost less than fresh. And they make it so easy to create fast dinners without having to make an extra trip to the store.
- If there is a thrift store bakery nearby, stock up on day-old whole-grain bread. Freeze loaves so you won't run out.

- Freeze bits of leftover canned ingredients like tomato paste and coconut milk.
- Try to find ethnic grocery stores in your area. Often, items that are expensive "specialty" foods in the regular grocery store are everyday food in Asian or Indian markets—and are much lower in price. This can be your ticket to saving on some of the more expensive vegan staples like soymilk, tahini, and tempeh.
- Visit www.localharvest.org/csa to find a community-supported agricultural group in your area, and talk to them to see if it would be a good fit for you. These programs allow you to buy shares in local farms—a good way to support small vegetable farmers and get quality organic produce—but depending on the specifics, they may or may not be a bargain.
- If you can't make everything from scratch, choose a few items that will save you real money and that you enjoy (or at least don't mind) doing. Homemade cakes and cookies made from scratch save lots of money. Making your own seitan from gluten flour is also a huge money saver; you can make a big batch every few months and freeze it. Other ways to save include homemade salad dressings (so easy to make—there is really never any excuse for buying them), peanut sauce, and hummus.
- If you have room—a sunny spot on a window sill—you can easily grow your own vegetables. Tomatoes, lettuce, and greens can all be grown in pots. Leafy greens like kale and Swiss chard will give you a harvest throughout the summer and well into the fall. If you like cooking with fresh herbs, a small herb garden—in the ground or in a pot—is a must since these foods are expensive at the grocery store.

All of the standard advice that works for budget-minded omnivores applies to vegan grocery shopping: Make a list and stick to it; buy in season; look for specials; avoid impulse purchases; and take advantage of bulk-food warehouse stores.

Don't Sweat the Small Stuff!

There are "hidden" animal ingredients in many foods. Even seemingly benign foods like white sugar and maple syrup—seemingly vegan—can be processed with animal ingredients, a fact that you won't see on their labels. Some food additives and food colors can be either animal- or plant-derived—and you have no way of knowing.

Should you care? Well, we don't think so. In fact, we're convinced that worrying about such things does more harm than good.

There is truly nothing to be gained by careful attention to this kind of detail in your diet. Avoiding these minute animal ingredients won't make your diet any healthier. Nor will it lessen animal suffering or help protect the environment, at least not in any meaningful way. The only thing it will do is make your vegan diet more restrictive, time-consuming, and difficult to follow. It's possible to get so bogged down in these details that you will simply find a vegan diet too laborious to follow.

Or you may be perfectly happy to put time and attention into seeking out and eliminating every last animal ingredient from your diet. While that is certainly your choice, it's important to think about how this impacts the general view of vegan diets. If others believe that this meticulous attention to detail is what a vegan diet means, they may be less inspired to eat this way themselves. If you want to have a wide impact, then it makes better sense to portray a vegan diet as something delicious, fun—and easy.

SOYFOODS PRIMER

You don't have to include soyfoods in your vegan diet, but they are so versatile and nutritious that many vegans find them indispensable. This group of foods has a long history of use in Asian countries, and they've been the focus of much research over the past couple of decades. We'll talk about nutrition, health, and safety issues related to soy in Chapter 15. Here is a quick rundown of the most commonly consumed soyfoods.

Soybeans

Soybeans are generally tan in color, but they can also be black or brown. They're a good source of protein, fiber, calcium, iron, and folate. Cooked soybeans have a flavor often described as "beany." It's a flavor that marries well with tomato sauces and spicy foods.

Edamame

These are soybeans that are harvested at about 75 percent maturity, while they are still green and have the nutrition of the whole soybean but with a milder flavor. In Japan, they are boiled in the pod and then served as a popular bar food (with beer). In the United States, you can find edamame already shelled in either the produce or frozen food section. Boil them for 15 minutes and eat as a vegetable or add them to grain salads. They're a good source of protein, fiber, and calcium.

Soynuts

Made from dry soybeans that have been soaked and then roasted, these are a good snack and a crunchy addition to salads. They are relatively high in fat and calories and are a good source of both protein and calcium.

Soymilk

This is the liquid expressed from soaked, pureed soybeans. It's a good source of protein and usually fortified with calcium, vitamin D, and vitamin B_{12}, and sometimes riboflavin. (Soymilk sold in Asian markets is often not fortified, so be certain to check labels.) Plain soymilk can stand in for cow's milk in just about any circumstance. Vanilla or chocolate soymilk can be used in smoothies or desserts.

Tofu

Made in the same way that cheese is made from cow's milk, tofu is produced by adding a curdling agent to soymilk. Though it is the source of many jokes in the Western world, tofu has a long and sacred history in the East. It's believed that the first tofu shops were located within the walls of Buddhist temples and the first tofu makers were monks. There is still a sense of the sacred attached to tofu and tofu-making in many parts of Asia today. It has been used for nearly 2,000 years in China and is a daily staple in most Asian households. Throughout Asia tofu is made fresh daily from soybeans in small shops and sold on the street by vendors.

If calcium sulfate is used in the manufacturing process, tofu is a good source of calcium. The protein content varies depending on processing, but some types, especially those that are more firm, are very high in protein.

Two properties give tofu great culinary versatility. First, its flavor is relatively bland. Second, it is a porous food that takes on the flavor of other foods and ingredients with ease. This explains why tofu is at home in spicy entrees or in creamy sweet desserts.

The key to success with tofu is to choose the right type for the job. If you are stir-frying chunks of tofu with veggies to serve over rice, choose firm tofu. Soft tofu is perfect to mash or puree as a filling for sandwiches or lasagna. And the tofu that is traditional to Japanese cooking, silken tofu, is a soft, custard-like food that can be blended or pureed for sauces, smoothies, or desserts. It is a great replacement for the cream in creamed soup recipes.

Frozen tofu takes on a chewy, spongy texture that makes it a useful meat substitute. Freeze it right in the unopened package. Then defrost, squeeze out the liquid, and chop or shred it.

Whole cookbooks are devoted to tofu, and we've included one of our favorites, *Tofu Cookery* by Louise Hagler, in the list of resources at the end of this book.

Okara

The word "kara" refers to the hull of the soybean, and the addition of "o" turns it into "honorable hull." This is the portion left behind when liquid is squeezed from the soaked soybean to make soymilk. It's high in protein and fiber and is sometimes used to give a protein boost to baked goods like muffins or cookies. In Japan, okara is sometimes sautéed with vegetables and served with rice. You may be able to find okara in natural foods stores, but the best place to track it down is in an Asian market.

FERMENTED SOYFOODS

Tempeh

In Indonesia, it's spelled *tempe*, and it is an ancient cultural staple of cooking in that part of the world. Today, tempeh-making is still a home-based art in which whole soybeans are treated with a "starter" and wrapped in banana leaves to ferment. Tempeh can be made from soybeans only or soybeans in combination with grains. The texture is tender and chewy, and the savory flavor is sometimes described as "yeasty" or "mushroom-like" or just indescribably delicious. In traditional meals, it's sautéed with vegetables and served over rice, sometimes with peanut sauce. Tempeh baked in barbecue sauce is a favorite with many vegans. Tempeh is a good source of protein, fiber, iron, and calcium. Contrary to popular opinion, however, it is not a good source of active vitamin B_{12}.

Miso

With a full-bodied flavor that is unmatched by any western condiment, miso captures the essence of Japanese cooking. This salty, fermented soybean paste (usually with addition of other beans or grains) comes in different colors—white, red, and brown—and the flavor varies greatly among types, with some being more fruity or wine-like than others. In fact, in Japan, miso production is regarded in a similar fashion to wine-making in other parts of the world. Miso is very high in sodium and a little goes a long way. Use it to make broths and sauces.

Natto

Made from whole soybeans fermented with a bacterial culture, natto has a distinctive aroma, flavor, and texture, which is often described as "gooey." It is a popular breakfast food in Japan, served with rice, but has not made its way onto many American menus. It may be the only known plant food that is high in vitamin K_2.

WESTERN SOYFOODS

Textured Vegetable Protein (TVP™)

Made from defatted soy flour, TVP is a dried granular product that can be rehydrated with boiling water and used in place of ground beef. Plain TVP tastes best when cooked in tomato sauce and is good for pasta dishes or chili. In her cookbook *Vegan Comfort Food*, Alicia Simpson recommends rehydrating 1 cup dry TVP with 1 cup of dark vegetable stock and 1 tablespoon of hickory liquid smoke. TVP is a very inexpensive source of protein with a long shelf life, and it's a good source of protein, fiber, and calcium.

Isolated Soy Protein

Many veggie meats use soy protein as a base. For those who are just making the transition to veganism or who are too busy to cook, veggie meats made from soy protein isolate can be life-savers.

Will You "Detox" When You Go Vegan?

One popular idea that circulates through vegan circles is that going vegan causes your body to "detox." The theory is that you'll have a few days or weeks of feeling awful as your body eliminates the toxic buildup from your not-so-healthy omnivore diet.

It's not true. For one thing, we are always detoxing. Normal everyday metabolism produces toxic compounds. The body has extensive systems in place—mostly involving the liver, kidneys, and lungs—that detoxify and/or excrete these compounds. It's true that a healthy lifestyle keeps these systems operating at optimal levels. But going vegan—even if you do it suddenly—does not produce a massive cleansing of toxins.

Likewise, there is no evidence that omnivores have physical addictions to animal foods. It may feel difficult to give up favorite foods like cheese and ice cream, but you won't suffer any physical withdrawal symptoms, unless you don't get enough protein or calories.

WHAT VEGANS EAT

Vegans love to say that giving up animal foods didn't shrink their food horizons; it expanded them. Is it true? We asked seventeen friends—health professionals, activists, athletes, cookbook authors, and a few teens—to tell us their favorite dinner that they cook at home. Their answers are proof positive that nobody knows good food like a vegan!

ERICA MEIER

Executive Director, Compassion Over Killing

▸ Quinoa topped with stir-fried vegetables, chick peas, and tempeh or veggie meats, like Field Roast or Gardein

"If I'm really feeling up for it, and have the ingredients, I might go all out and make the recipe for Pineapple Cashew Quinoa stir-fry from the cookbook *Veganomicon*. (We love quinoa, what can I say?)"

INGRID NEWKIRK

President of People for the Ethical Treatment of Animals

▸ English Stew

"This lasts for days and changes in that time. I used to use beef bones in the old days, which makes me feel so sick to think of them clanging around in the bottom of the pot. I instantly weaned from that rich, bloody flavor by adding a couple of tablespoons of Marmite or Vegemite but now love to add a small can of medium-hot Mexican green chili peppers and tomatoes at the end.

I use a base of Manischewitz dry minestrone soup mix and just shove in any fresh and/or frozen veggies, usually potatoes, broccoli, a bag of mixed peas, carrots, tomatoes, or cauliflower, but really any vegetables, some garlic or not, some onion for sure, and bring it to the boil and then let it simmer. I am Phyllis Diller in the kitchen—shouldn't be there. But I love this, can thermos it to work, take it on the train, pour it over rice, leave the Mex spice bits out, and add lentils or more peas or corn, and then before it all disappears, spice it up. Love it with a warm baguette, with crackers or croutons, on toast or rice. And my old dog, Ms. Bea, worshipped it. It's dirt cheap too."

LOUISE HAGLER

The Soybean Queen, cookbook author and soybean pioneer

Louise, who works with the hunger relief organization Plenty International, says that this menu is a hit in her nutrition classes in Mexico.

▸ Chewy Tofu Nuggets (from the twenty-fifth anniversary edition of *Tofu Cookery*) rolled up in corn tortillas with sautéed Swiss chard and caramelized onions

REED MANGELS, PHD, RD

Co-author of the American Dietetic Association's Position on Vegetarian Diets; Lecturer, Nutrition Department, University of Massachusetts; and Nutrition Advisor to the Vegetarian Resource Group

Reed says that sushi is a meal she doesn't make very often, because it's time-consuming, but both of her teenage daughters, Leah and Sarah, choose it as a favorite.

....

"I cook the rice (using the Nori-Maki Sushi recipe and instructions in Nava Atlas's *Vegetarian Celebrations*) and prepare bowls of fillings. Everyone makes his or her favorite filling combination, rolls the sushi, and we slice it. Here are some favorite fillings:

▸ Baked tofu
▸ Avocado strips

- ▶ Cucumber strips
- ▶ Carrot strips
- ▶ Peas
- ▶ Red pepper strips
- ▶ Steamed zucchini strips
- ▶ Asparagus

"We often have peanut sauce and soy sauce for dipping the sushi. I usually make a stir-fry using whatever vegetables are around. Watermelon slices in summer or chocolate chip cookies from *Joy of Vegan Baking* for dessert."

JON CAMP

Director of Outreach for Vegan Outreach

Jon is always on the road, so we let him share a restaurant meal instead of one that he cooks at home.

....

"My favorite meal is the vegetarian platter from Ethiopian restaurants. You get to choose from a number of items. I opt for split peas, collard greens, sliced cabbage with carrots, red lentils, and string beans with potatoes. Additionally, various places throughout the United States offer tofu dishes and/or mock meats. All of these selections are cooked in sauces teeming with garlic, ginger, onions, etc. No silverware is required; you scoop the food up with *injera*, a slightly spongy bread made from teff flour. Ethiopian restaurants can be found in virtually every major metropolitan region throughout the country. In short, it is the stuff of the gods."

BRYANNA CLARK GROGAN

Cookbook author and blogger at
www.veganfeastkitchen.blogspot.com

Bryanna has been studying food and cooking for forty years and has written eight vegan cookbooks. Her favorite menu is the following Italian-style autumn dinner. The recipes are all from her cookbooks *Nonna's Italian Kitchen* and *World Vegan Feast.*

▸ Vegan Italian Cream of Cabbage Soup (*Passato di Cavalo*)
▸ Lentil and Rapini Stew with Spicy Vegan Italian Sausage (using Field Roast or Tofurky sausages)
▸ Homemade No-Knead Crusty Artisan Bread
▸ Sicilian Style Fennel and Orange Salad (mixed greens, sliced oranges, fennel, red onion, black olives, and red wine vinaigrette)
▸ Crostata di Pere (Italian pear tart in a low-fat corn pastry)
▸ Homemade Almond Cream Whipped Topping (or commercial vegan vanilla ice cream)

SCOTT SPITZ

Competitive distance runner and blogger at
http://runvegan.wordpress.com/

"We make awesome food on a consistent basis in this household! We are big fans of combining foods to make one big meal (stir-fry, pasta with peanut sauce and veggies, etc.). But this is a favorite dinner with vegetables on the side."

▸ BBQ tempeh on a bed of brown rice and steamed kale
▸ A side of sweet potatoes
▸ Apple crisp for dessert

JANE VELEZ-MITCHELL

*Newscaster and host of
CNN's* Issues with Jane Velez-Mitchell

"My favorite meal is kasha with soy butter. Kasha is a warm cereal eaten in Eastern Europe. It's generally made of buckwheat groats. That may not sound tasty but it is. It will make you as strong as a horse! Kasha is so simple to make: Just get some from your local health food store or coop, add some water, and turn up the flame on your burner. Voila! Add soy butter to taste. It is hearty, nutritious, and delicious! FYI, this is one of the oldest porridge-style meals in Eastern Europe, so get back to basics and try some kasha!"

SAM STAHLER

*Twelve-year-old son of Debra Wasserman and Charles Stahler,
co-founders of the Vegetarian Resource Group*

Sam gave us two menus and his mom said that he makes these himself.

▸ For breakfast: Scrambled tofu with onion, carrots, soyrizo or chopped veggie "bacon," seasoned with pepper, turmeric, and cayenne and served with fortified orange juice
▸ For dinner: Canned Amy's vegan chili (spicy only!) and rice with broccoli or kale

ISA CHANDRA MOSKOWITZ

Author of cookbooks including the acclaimed Veganomicon

- Cauliflower mashed potatoes
- Mushroom gravy
- Garlicky sautéed Swiss shard
- Baked tempeh

PAUL SHAPIRO

*Senior Director, The Humane Society
of the United States' Factory Farming Campaign*

- Burrito made from whole-wheat tortilla with greens, quinoa, and beans
- Mashed sweet potatoes
- Fruit smoothie

BRUCE FRIEDRICH
AND ALKA CHANDNA

People for the Ethical Treatment of Animals

Indian dinner combination including:

- Chana masala (spicy chickpeas)
- Aloo gobi (potatoes and cauliflower)
- Achar (Indian pickles)

NATHAN RUNKLE

Founder and Executive Director of Mercy For Animals

▶ Vegan Reuben Sandwich: sliced seitan, onions, peppers, sauerkraut, vegan Thousand Island dressing, and Daiya cheese served on marbled rye
▶ Raw lemon coconut cheesecake for dessert

MATT BALL

Co-founder of Vegan Outreach

▶ Taco made with Gimme Lean, ground-beef style, and Ortega taco seasoning
▶ Topped with refried beans, Daiya cheese, Tofutti sour cream, and hot sauce
▶ Spanish rice

NEAL BARNARD, MD

*President and founder of the
Physicians Committee for Responsible Medicine*

▶ Green salad with light vinaigrette
▶ Capellini (angel hair pasta) with arrabbiata sauce
▶ Broccoli, spinach, and carrots, all steamed and served with lemon wedges

SUE HAVALA-HOBBS, DPH, RD

Director, Doctoral Program in Health Leadership,
School of Public Health, University of North Carolina;
and co-author of the American Dietetic Association's 1988
and 1993 Position on Vegetarian Diets

▶ Kale cooked with soy-ginger sauce, tempeh cubes, and toasted pine nuts over steamed rice
▶ Steamed carrots
▶ Whole-grain dinner roll
▶ Baked apple with vanilla soy yogurt

MELANIE JOY, PHD

Psychologist and author of
Why We Love Dogs, Eat Pigs and Wear Cows

▶ Pizza with whole-wheat crust (from Trader Joe's) topped with organic tomato sauce with crushed garlic, Field Roast apple sage sausage, baby spinach, black olives, and Daiya cheese
▶ Mesclun mix salad with goddess dressing or sautéed kale with slivered garlic and toasted almonds
▶ Sliced Asian pear sprinkled with cinnamon for dessert

CHAPTER 9

A HEALTHY START
Vegan Diets in Pregnancy and Breast-Feeding

Family members, friends, and even your health-care provider might express surprise and concern at the idea of a vegan pregnancy. But vegan diets can easily meet the nutritional needs of you and your growing baby. The proof comes from a 1987 study of 775 women living on the Farm, a vegan community in Tennessee.[1] The researchers looked at weight gain in pregnant women and birth weights of their babies—two important measures of a healthy pregnancy. They found that the women's vegan diets had no effect on the birth weights of their babies and that their own weight gain during pregnancy was adequate. In fact, these women actually gained a little bit more than women in the general meat-eating population. And the longer they had been vegan, the better their weight gain.

One other finding was surprising: Preeclampsia, a potential complication of pregnancy that occurs in 5 to 10 percent of pregnant women, was nearly nonexistent among vegan pregnant women living on the Farm. Along with another smaller study, these findings give reassurance that vegan diets are safe and healthy for pregnancy.

In some studies of women following very restrictive diets, particularly macrobiotic diets, infants sometimes had lower birth weights. In these cases, it wasn't a vegan diet that was to blame. Rather, the diets at issue were too low in fat and calories. It's important to note that the findings about poor pregnancy outcomes are from older studies when vegans had less access to nutrition information and a variety of vegan foods. That's all changed dramatically in the past several decades, and today it's easier than ever to plan a healthy vegan pregnancy.

GETTING ENOUGH CALORIES

Although adequate weight gain is important for a healthy vegan pregnancy, eating for two doesn't mean eating twice as many calories. On average, pregnant women need an extra 340 calories per day during the second trimester and 450 extra calories during the last three months of pregnancy. But needs for certain nutrients increase by as much as 50 percent, so packing a lot of good nutrition into that little bit of extra food is important.

Pregnant women can follow the vegan food guide in Chapter 7 with just a few adjustments that we've shown in the Modified Food Guide for Pregnancy and Breast-feeding on page 140. An added serving each of whole grains and leafy green vegetables and two additional servings of protein-rich foods (legumes, nuts, and soyfoods) will give you needed calories and help meet nutrient needs during the second trimester. During the last trimester, when your baby is growing fastest, add one more serving of either whole grains or legumes/soyfoods.

Calorie-counting during pregnancy isn't an exact science, but your health-care provider will help you stay on track by monitoring your weight gain. Poor weight gain during pregnancy is associated with low-birth-weight babies, who are at risk for health problems.

NUTRITION CONSIDERATIONS IN VEGAN PREGNANCY

The table on page 139 shows changes in nutrient needs for pregnant and nursing women.

Protein needs increase by almost 50 percent in pregnancy. Most non-pregnant omnivore women consume enough protein to meet the needs of pregnancy, but that may not be true of all vegan women. It isn't difficult to get enough, but it's important to make sure you are including at least five to six servings of protein-rich foods from the food guide in your daily menus.

Iron absorption—especially of the nonheme iron found in plant foods—increases significantly during pregnancy while the lack of menstruation reduces iron losses. Even so, iron requirements nearly double during pregnancy. Some of the increased iron requirement is due to the manufacture of red blood cells in the growing fetus, but most of it is needed to support the expansion of the mother's blood volume during pregnancy. Theoretically, vegans could be at higher risk for iron deficiency in pregnancy, but the truth is that all women are at risk. It's difficult to plan diets for either vegans or omnivores that meet iron needs of pregnancy. For that reason, iron supplements are almost always recommended for pregnant women.

Pregnant women typically have zinc intakes that are lower than recommendations, unless they are taking supplements. The benefits of zinc supplements in pregnancy aren't known, but they may be beneficial for pregnant vegans since zinc absorption from plant foods is lower than from meat.

Vitamin D requirements don't change with pregnancy, but getting enough is important for both the mother's and baby's health. With the exception of vitamin B_{12} and iron and—depending on your diet—possibly vitamin D and iodine, it is possible to meet all of the nutrient needs of pregnancy on a vegan diet without the use of supplements. But most health professionals recommend a prenatal multivitamin and mineral supplement, particularly one that includes iron and folate, as sensible insurance for both vegan and omnivore women.

Pregnant vegetarians have lower blood levels of DHA (the long-chain omega-3 fatty acid) than pregnant nonvegetarians.[2] We don't know whether that's a problem, but there is some evidence that DHA intake during pregnancy and breast-feeding improves visual acuity and brain function in the infant. Experts recommend that pregnant women consume 300 milligrams of DHA per day, so we recommend DHA algae-derived supplements for vegans.

Here are some tips for a healthy vegan pregnancy:

- If you are planning a pregnancy, now is the time to take a good look at your eating habits. Healthy nutrition in the early weeks of pregnancy—often before a woman knows that she is pregnant—is important. Make sure your diet includes plenty of foods that are rich in the B-vitamin folic acid. Good sources are legumes and leafy green vegetables. Think about cutting alcohol out of your diet, too, if there is any chance you might become pregnant, and if you are a coffee drinker, now is the time to cut back.

- Talk to your health-care provider about your weight-gain goals. If you have trouble gaining weight, emphasize foods with a little more fat, such as tofu, nut butters, and avocados.

- Use the Modified Vegan Food Guide for Pregnancy and Breast-feeding on page 140 in making daily food choices.

- Protein needs go up by about 25 grams beginning with the second trimester. It's not difficult to meet those needs on a vegan diet, but it might require extra attention. Take a look at the list of protein-rich foods in Chapter 2. Aim for at least 15 to 20 grams of protein in each meal and choose a few protein-rich snacks as well.

- Eat plenty of iron-rich foods and include a good source of vitamin C at every meal to boost absorption. Most health-care professionals recommend iron supplements for all pregnant women. This can be especially helpful for vegans since iron needs are higher for those on plant-based diets.

- Eat plenty of foods high in the B-vitamin folic acid. If you don't typically use refined enriched grain products, which are fortified with folic acid, make sure you are consuming plenty of folic acid–rich foods if there is a possibility you could become pregnant. Vegans generally have higher intakes of folic acid than omnivores, but they still aren't high enough to meet pregnancy needs. A prenatal supplement that contains folic acid is a wise choice for all pregnant women.

- Some pregnant vegans don't meet requirements for zinc, a nutrient that can fall short even in well-planned vegan diets. Be sure to include whole grains, legumes, and a serving or two of nuts or seeds in your meals. A supplement providing 15 to 25 milligrams of zinc can be a good choice for pregnant vegans. It should also supply 2 milligrams of copper since zinc can lower copper absorption.

- Because calcium absorption is more efficient during pregnancy, pregnant women don't have increased needs for this nutrient. It's important to get enough, though, so make sure you emphasize foods that are calcium-rich. Make it a daily habit to eat a serving or two of leafy green vegetables and choose calcium-fortified soymilk and orange juice. Recommendations for calcium intake are 1,000 milligrams per day.

- Supplement daily with vitamin B_{12} and, unless you are absolutely certain that you are getting adequate sun exposure, take a supplement of vitamin D as well.

- Although it is usually called morning sickness, nausea associated with early pregnancy can occur at any time of day. In addition to being unpleasant, nausea can keep you from eating healthfully. Here are a few tips to help you deal with pregnancy-induced nausea:

  ▸ Eat frequent small meals since an empty stomach can make nausea worse. (Small meals can also help with heartburn, which can be a problem for some pregnant women.)

  ▸ Eat something immediately upon waking, when your stomach is likely to be empty. Keep crackers or raisins or whatever appeals to you on the bedside table.

  ▸ Avoid liquids with meals if you find that this increases your nausea.

  ▸ Identify healthy foods that are less likely to make you feel sick. You'll need to follow your own instincts, but good choices to consider include whole-grain breads, dry cereals, cooked or dried fruits, and white or sweet potatoes. Try adding small pieces of vegetables and tofu to miso soup to make them saltier and easier on your stomach.

VEGAN NUTRITION FOR NURSING MOMS

The rate of breast-feeding is higher among vegan mothers than in the general population. And that's nice for their babies since breast milk is the ideal food for infants. Ideally, babies should be fed human milk for at least the first year of their lives and preferably throughout the second year as well.

Nursing mothers need extra calories for the process of synthesizing milk and to provide the calories that babies need for growth. Energy needs, therefore, are higher during lactation than in pregnancy. If you have post-pregnancy pounds to drop, a small reduction in calories can usually produce a gradual weight loss while still maintaining adequate milk volume. Don't decrease calories too much, though, as it can cause the milk supply to decrease as well. Drinking plenty of fluids is also important for producing adequate milk.

Needs for some nutrients go up slightly, so keeping the emphasis on nutrient-rich foods is as important as ever. (One exception is iron: Since breast-feeding women don't menstruate, iron needs drop to very low levels during lactation.) Diet affects the levels of all of the vitamins in breast milk as well as the type of fat.

The two nutrients that require the most attention in vegan diets are ones that nutrition-savvy vegans are already focusing on—vitamin D and vitamin B_{12}. Deficiencies of these nutrients have been seen in babies whose mothers didn't follow recommended guidelines and they can cause serious problems. Nursing women should consume a daily vitamin B_{12} supplement. We also recommend continuing with a DHA supplement since one study showed that the milk of vegan women is lower in this nutrient than that of omnivores.[3]

Many women continue with a prenatal supplement for the first few months of breast-feeding (but without the extra iron). And the American Academy of Pediatrics recommends vitamin D supplements for all breast-fed infants (not just those in vegan families).

NUTRIENT RECOMMENDATIONS FOR NONPREGNANT, PREGNANT, AND BREAST-FEEDING WOMEN

Nutrient	Non-pregnant	Pregnant	Breast-feeding
Protein (g)*	46	71	71
Thiamin (mg)	1.1	1.4	1.4
Riboflavin (mg)	1.1	1.4	1.6
Niacin (mg)	14	18	17
Vitamin B$_6$ (mg)	1.3	1.9	2.0
Folic acid (µg)	400	600	500
Vitamin B$_{12}$ (µg)	2.4	2.6	2.8
Vitamin C (mg)	75	85	120
Vitamin A (µg)	700	770	1,300
Vitamin D (IU)	600	600	600
Vitamin E (mg)	15	15	19
Vitamin K (µg)	90	90	90
Calcium (mg)	1,000	1,000	1,000
Iodine (µg)	150	220	290
Iron (mg**)	18	27	9
Magnesium (mg)	310–320	350–360	310–320
Phosphorus (mg)	700	700	700
Selenium (µg)	55	60	70
Zinc (mg)***	8	11	12

*Protein needs may be slightly higher for pregnant vegans. Use the guidelines in Chapter 2 to calculate your pre-pregnancy protein requirements and then add 25 to 28 extra grams of protein for pregnancy.
** Iron recommendations for vegetarians and vegans are 1.8 times higher than this.
***Zinc requirements for some vegans could be as much as 50 percent higher.

MODIFIED FOOD GUIDE FOR PREGNANCY AND BREAST-FEEDING

These are minimum servings and should be used as a general guide. Some women will need more than this to support adequate weight gain.

Food group	Servings per day during pregnancy	Servings per day while breast-feeding
Grains and starchy vegetables	6–7	6–7
Legumes and soyfoods	5–6	6
Nuts	2	2
Vegetables	5 (include at least one leafy green vegetable)	5
Fruits	2	2
Fats	3	3
Calcium-rich foods	8	8

Supplements for pregnant vegans:

- A chewable or sublingual vitamin B_{12} supplement. Follow the guidelines in Chapter 3. Don't rely on a multivitamin supplement for this unless it is chewable.
- Prenatal supplement that provides folic acid, zinc, iron, and copper.
- A calcium supplement if you feel you are falling short of the 1,000 milligrams of calcium recommended during pregnancy.
- 300 milligrams of DHA from algae.
- 150 micrograms of iodine (which may already be included in your prenatal supplement).
- 600 to 1,000 IU vitamin D unless you are certain that you have adequate sun exposure.

Supplements for breastfeeding vegans:

- A chewable or sublingual vitamin B_{12} supplement
- 300 milligrams of DHA
- 150 micrograms of iodine

SAMPLE MENUS

You may very well feel like cooking up a storm during and after your pregnancy. But just in case you don't have the time or energy for much food prep, we've kept things simple with these sample menus. They are meant to illustrate the ease of planning healthy vegan menus without fuss. These menus utilize six mini-meals, which can be helpful with managing heartburn and nausea.

Sample Menu for Pregnancy

Breakfast
- 1 cup fortified breakfast cereal
- 1 cup fortified soymilk
- Banana

Snack
- ¼ cup almonds
- Raw vegetables

Lunch
- Miso soup with ½ cup tofu and 1 cup cooked kale or collards
- Serving of whole-grain crackers

Snack
- Whole-grain bread with ½ cup hummus
- ½ cup fortified orange juice

Dinner
- 1 cup brown rice
- ½ cup baked beans
- 1 cup steamed vegetables sautéed in 2 teaspoons canola oil

Snack
- ½ whole-grain English muffin with 2 tablespoons almond butter
- 1 cup fortified soymilk

Sample Menu for Breast-Feeding

Breakfast

▸ ½ cup scrambled tofu cooked in 1 teaspoon canola oil
▸ 1 slice whole-wheat toast with 1 teaspoon margarine
▸ 1 cup calcium-fortified orange juice

Snack

▸ ½ cup grapes
▸ Serving of whole-grain crackers with 2 tablespoons almond butter

Lunch

▸ Veggie burger
▸ Whole-wheat hamburger roll
▸ Slice tomato and lettuce
▸ Broccoli salad with ½ tablespoon vegan mayonnaise

Snack

▸ Small bran muffin
▸ 1 cup fortified soymilk

Dinner

▸ 1 cup lentil soup
▸ 1 cup steamed collards
▸ Green salad with dressing
▸ Whole-wheat dinner roll
▸ Snack

Smoothie

▸ ½ cup fortified soymilk
▸ ½ cup frozen fruit
▸ ¼ banana
▸ 1 teaspoon ground flaxseed

CHAPTER 10

RAISING VEGAN CHILDREN AND TEENS

INFANTS

Even the most confident vegan adults might feel a little nervous about a vegan diet for their newborn baby. Infants typically triple their weight in the first year of life and need enough nutritious food to see them through this early growth spurt. Can a vegan diet satisfy their needs?

During the first months of a baby's life, this isn't even an issue. All infants start out as vegetarians. Or, to be more correct, they begin their lives as "lactarians." For the first four months or so, infants don't need anything other than breast milk. It's the perfect, complete food for a newborn. Unless they are given B_{12} supplements (needed only if the mom's diet is inadequate), the diets of vegan babies are exactly the same as infants in omnivore families until they are around seven months old.

The First Four Months

For the first four to six months of life, babies don't need—and shouldn't have—anything other than breast milk (or infant formula). They don't need any solid foods during this time, and certain vegetables can be dangerous to very young infants.

Between the ages of four and six months, babies start to show that they are ready for solid foods. One sign of readiness is the ability to sit up and maintain balance. Another is the ability to use the tongue to move food to the back of the mouth for swallowing. Your pediatrician will help you decide when your baby is ready for solid foods, but all babies should start having some solid foods no later than six months of age.[1]

First Solid Food Adventure: Cereal

"Solid" is a bit of an overstatement for the first non-milk foods a baby eats. They are more like thick liquids—fed from a spoon, not a bottle.

The first food for an infant is usually an iron-fortified infant rice cereal mixed with breast milk or infant formula. There isn't anything wrong with other choices, but rice cereal is easily digested and unlikely to cause allergies. Once a baby is used to cereal and eating around ⅓ cup per day, begin to introduce mashed fruits and vegetables like applesauce, banana, pureed peaches or pears, strained white and sweet potatoes, carrots, green beans, and avocado.

During this period, breast milk or soy formula continues to play a major role in your baby's diet and will be a part of the menu until at least the first birthday. Breast milk or infant formula is especially important for providing zinc, which can otherwise be low in a vegan infant's diet. Even after your baby starts to consume solid foods, he or she needs either breast milk or a commercial infant formula. Regular soymilk should never be offered to babies before the first birthday because, like cow's milk, it is a poor fit for an infant's nutritional needs. Be sure to read "When Breast-Feeding Isn't an Option" on page 147.

First Protein Foods

At around seven months, your baby will be ready to drink apple juice from a cup and explore protein-rich foods. This is when the diet of a baby in a vegan household starts to look a little bit different from that of other infants. First protein-rich foods for vegan infants include legumes (cook them thoroughly and puree them), well-mashed tofu, and soy yogurt. This is a good time to start introducing vegetables with a stronger flavor like kale and collards. You can temper their flavors by pureeing them with bland or sweet foods like applesauce, tofu, or avocado.

Infants are usually ready for finger foods, like chunks of tofu or meat analogs, bread, and crackers, at ten months, and by the first birthday they can have nut butters or tahini spread thinly on crackers.

A few things to keep in mind for vegan babies:

- Talk to your pediatrician about supplements. Vitamin D is usually recommended for breast-fed infants in both vegan and omnivore families. Iron is sometimes recommended beginning at around four months, but that will depend on other foods in your baby's diet. Breast-fed vegan infants need vitamin B_{12} supplements only if the mother's diet isn't adequate. The table on page 146 shows suggested supplements for breast-fed vegan infants.
- When your baby is ready for solid foods, introduce them one at a time, offering one new food every three to four days. This makes it easy to identify any food allergies right away.
- Never give babies unpasteurized juice or cider, or any kind of corn syrup or honey, all of which can cause serious illness.
- Be careful not to overdo it with juices. Too much juice can displace other nutritious foods in a baby's diet and can also cause diarrhea. Limit your infant to 6 ounces of juice per day and avoid juices with added sweeteners.
- Don't give a baby any milk other than breast milk or infant formula before the first birthday. Regular soy, rice, hemp, and almond milks don't have the right balance of nutrients for infants and shouldn't be offered until your baby is a year old (these milks can, however, be used in small amounts in food preparation).
- Don't offer foods that can cause choking like whole tofu hotdogs, popcorn, nuts, hard candies and grapes. Don't offer infants nut and seed butters by the spoonful or spread too thickly on bread.
- Don't salt or sweeten foods.

	DAILY SUPPLEMENTS FOR BREAST-FED VEGAN BABIES	
Nutrient	*Birth to 6 months*	*6 to 12 months*
Vitamin D	400 IU (10 micrograms)	400 IU (10 microgram)
Vitamin B$_{12}$	0.4 micrograms only if the mother doesn't have a reliable B$_{12}$ intake	0.5 micrograms only if the mother doesn't have a reliable B$_{12}$ intake
Iron	1 milligram per kilogram (0.45 milligrams per pound) of body weight beginning at four months	1 milligram per kilogram (0.45 milligrams per pound) of body weight unless infant is consuming sufficient iron from solid foods
Fluoride		0.25 milligrams if water contains less than 0.3 parts per million fluoride

Adapted from A. R. Mangels and V. Messina, "Considerations in Planning Vegan Diets: Infants," *Journal of the American Dietetic Association.*[2]

THE FIRST BIRTHDAY AND BEYOND: VEGAN TODDLERS

After the mad growth spurt and enthusiastic appetite of the first twelve months, things begin to slow down. Toddlers can have sluggish appetites, and children aren't known for their adventurous eating habits at this stage. Picky and sometimes quirky eating behavior can make it difficult to get toddlers and preschoolers to eat anything at all, let alone to try new foods.

Full-fat fortified soymilk can be introduced to a baby on the first birthday. Avoid using other milks made from rice, almonds, hemp, coconut, or oats as the main beverage, since they are too low in protein (and calories) for young children. If your child is a slow grower or you aren't certain that his or her diet is high enough in zinc, it might be wise to continue with either breast-feeding or soy infant formula for a while.

The food guide on page 149 and table of suggested supplements on page 159 will help you plan healthy meals for toddlers. Don't worry if

When Breast-Feeding Isn't an Option

For a number of reasons, breast milk is the optimal food for babies, and most vegans choose it for their newest family members. Breast milk provides a nutrient balance that is close to ideal for growing infants. It also contains unique immune factors and reduces the risk for allergies. Infants don't need any food other than breast milk for the first four to six months of life, and ideally they should continue to receive it until at least the first birthday or preferably the second.

But sometimes breast-feeding isn't an option. If you are unable to breast-feed or you need to decrease or stop nursing, soy infant formula supports normal growth and development in babies.[3] These formulas are not 100 percent vegan since they contain vitamin D derived from animals, but they are as close as we can get to a healthy vegan choice.

Infants should never be given homemade formulas and they should never be given regular soymilk. In the rare cases where vegan infants have suffered from malnutrition, it's because they were being fed homemade formulas or did not receive adequate supplements of vitamin B_{12} and vitamin D. Because babies have very specific nutritional needs, it's essential to use only commercial infant formulas which are manufactured to meet those needs.

your child doesn't eat exactly this way every single day. Two or three days of nothing but peanut butter and banana sandwiches never hurt anyone—not even a three-year-old. And getting children to eat healthful foods like vegetables isn't a vegan problem; it's a universal problem for parents of young children.

If you feel like your little one isn't eating enough, focus on higher-calorie foods that he or she enjoys, such as avocado, nut butters, and tofu. Don't overdo it with fiber, which can fill up small stomachs. Avoid foods like bran cereal, which are very high in fiber. While it's good to serve mostly whole grains, it's also okay to include some refined grains, such as regular pasta, in a toddler's diet. Low-fat diets can make it very difficult for young children to meet calorie needs, so don't skimp on fat in your child's diet. Toddlers and preschoolers will benefit from several small meals throughout the day; nutritious snacks are especially important for this age group.

As you explore new foods with your child, it's important to keep an open mind. You'll hear over and over again: Oh, no three-year-old will eat asparagus! Well, guess what? Some three-year-olds do. He may indeed be the rare three-year-old, but he may also be yours! So don't second-guess what your child will or won't eat based on what *most* kids prefer. After all, toddlers in Mexico eat pinto beans, and two-year-old Chinese kids dine happily on tofu.

Research shows that it takes as many as ten exposures to a new food before a young child will try it, so be persistent. If your child turns her nose up at baked beans, serve them again, in a different type of meal, after a week or so. And again. And again. It can help to serve new foods in small amounts alongside foods that are already familiar, and it's also important for children to observe you enjoying the food you're introducing.

Children are more likely to try foods that are easy to eat and that they can pick up with their fingers. If a toddler or preschooler is going through a picky phase and refuses to eat a variety of foods, it's okay to sneak foods into the diet any way you can. Your child may turn up his nose at a glass of soymilk but might be perfectly content to consume it when it's used to make mashed potatoes, pancakes, or chocolate pudding. Getting vegetables into the diet of a young vegan can be more of a challenge. Here are ideas that parents have found helpful:

- Finely chop leafy green vegetables and add to spaghetti sauce.
- Mix chopped raw kale, collards, or broccoli with rice and roll up in a tortilla.
- Add raw kale to fruit smoothies.
- Mix finely chopped carrots, sweet red peppers, and broccoli into vegan cream cheese, roll it up in a soft tortilla, and slice into colorful pinwheels.

FOOD GUIDE FOR VEGAN TODDLERS, AGES ONE TO THREE

Food group	Servings per day	Serving sizes
Grains	6 or more	½–1 slice bread; ¼–½ cup cooked cereal, grain, or pasta; ½–1 cup ready-to-eat cereal
Legumes, nuts, and other protein-rich foods	2 or more (vegan children should include at least 1 serving per day of nuts or seeds or 1 full-fat soy product)	¼–½ cup cooked beans, tofu, tempeh, or textured vegetable protein; 1 ounce meat analog; 1–2 tablespoons nuts, seeds, or nut or seed butter
Vegetables	2 or more	½–1 cup raw
Fruits	3 or more	¼–½ cup canned; ½ cup juice; ½ medium piece of fruit
Fats	3–4	1 teaspoon margarine or oil
Fortified soymilk or breast milk	3	1 cup

Adapted from V. Messina and A. R. Mangels, "Considerations in Planning Vegan Diets: Children," *Journal of the American Dietetic Association.*[4]

- Use raw vegetables to make salads in the shape of animals, or use cookie cutters to make fun-shaped sandwiches.
- Temper the strong flavor of kale and collards by blending them with bland foods such as avocado, tofu, or tofu cream cheese.

Valuable Foods for Vegan Children

Although there is no requirement for any type of milk in a child's diet, fortified soymilk can make it easier for vegan children to satisfy their nutrient needs. Other fortified milks, such as almond, oat, rice, or hemp milk, can be used in moderation, but since they are low in protein, they can displace protein-rich foods from the diet.

Nuts and seeds and the butters made from them can also be important in the diets of young children since they are energy and nutrient-rich. Red Star–brand Vegetarian Support Formula nutritional yeast is a

Sample Menu for Toddler

BREAKFAST
- ½ cup whole-grain ready-to-eat cereal
- 1 cup fortified soymilk
- ½ banana

SNACK
- ½ cup stewed dried apricots

LUNCH
- ¼ cup hummus
- 1 small (4-inch) pita
- ½ cup shredded carrot salad with ½ tablespoon vegan mayonnaise
- ½ cup calcium-fortified apple juice

SNACK
- ½ slice bread
- 1 tablespoon peanut butter
- 1 cup fortified soymilk

DINNER
- 3 pasta shells stuffed with ¼ cup pureed soft tofu
- ¼ cup steamed broccoli with 1 teaspoon margarine
- ¼ cup butternut squash topped with 1 teaspoon brown sugar

SNACK
- 1 cup fortified soymilk
- 1 graham cracker

good source of B vitamins, including vitamin B_{12}. Add nutritional yeast to bean dishes, veggie burgers, scrambled tofu, or mashed potatoes.

Blackstrap molasses (but not regular molasses) is a great source of calcium and iron. It has a strong taste and is likely to be more acceptable to children when mixed into other foods like smoothies, baked beans, or baked treats. It can also be mixed into peanut or almond butter and spread on crackers or bread.

ON THEIR OWN: VEGAN SCHOOL-AGE CHILDREN

The school years bring a new set of challenges as children encounter school lunches, birthday parties at McDonald's, and overnights with friends. Some kids may be savvy to the ways of the meat-eating world; others may have had less exposure to the idea that their diets are "different."

Will your child's vegan habits follow him as he heads out the door? Parents are likely to be faced with a series of decisions about this—personal decisions with no right or wrong answer. Some parents believe that a 100 percent vegan approach is most in line with their family's values and least likely to be confusing to a child. Others might allow some flexibility in certain social situations. Regardless, as children grow older, there will be times when parents no longer have control over what goes into their young ones' stomachs.

At home, however, parents can provide well-balanced vegan meals by following the food guide in Chapter 7 with some modifications to the number of servings as we've shown on page 158.

In public schools, cafeterias are unlikely to have regular vegan choices, and lunches brought from home are usually the best option. Try a laptop lunch box, based on the Japanese bento box. With compartments for four or five different foods, it allows you to create lunches with variety and fun appeal.

VEGAN TEENS

Growth during the teen years is faster than at any other time except for infancy. Needs increase dramatically for calories, protein, calcium and—for girls—iron. Meeting these needs can be a challenge since teens eat many meals on the go or on their own, and nutrition isn't

BROWN BAG OR LAPTOP LUNCHES
FOR VEGAN SCHOOLCHILDREN

Ideas for sandwiches or wraps
- Hummus with chopped apples
- Almond butter with shredded carrots
- Tofu salad with vegan mayonnaise and chopped celery
- Vegan cheese, avocado, and veggies
- Chopped chickpea salad with vegan mayonnaise
- Peanut butter and apple slices
- White beans pureed with cooked carrots and mixed with chopped apples and walnuts
- Avocado blended with shredded vegetables
- Potato salad made with cooked potatoes, chopped carrots, and tahini dressing
- Crumbled tofu, shredded raw cabbage, and peanut butter dressing
- Lentils with corn and sunflower seeds
- Vegan turkey and cheese
- Pinwheels: chopped vegetables and vegan cream cheese rolled in a whole-wheat flour tortilla and sliced into rounds

In the thermos
- Canned or homemade vegetarian chili
- Vegetable soup
- Beans and franks: vegetarian baked beans with tofu hotdogs

On the side:
- Fresh fruit
- Raw vegetables with tahini or tofu dip
- Baked tortilla chips
- Pasta or rice salad
- Bagel chips
- Vegetarian sushi

Sweet treats:
- Peanut butter or oatmeal cookies
- Soy or coconut yogurt
- Dried fruit or trail mix
- Graham crackers
- Granola bars
- Pitted dates rolled in shredded coconut or finely chopped nuts
- Nutty fruit bites: dried fruit, nuts, and peanut butter blended in a food processor and rolled into bite-sized balls

always a high priority. Many adolescents, vegan or not, fail to get enough calcium and iron. Diets often are too high in fat and sugar and low in fiber.

Teens raised in vegan households might have an edge over omnivore teens since they are likely to be familiar with a wide range of healthy plant foods. On the other hand, vegan teens may have to pay even more attention to calcium and iron than their omnivore peers. The biggest challenge faces teenagers in omnivore families who have chosen to adopt a vegan diet on their own. In that case, it's important for parents to offer support by learning about vegan diets and making sure the kitchen is well-stocked with lots of vegan foods.

The food guide on page 158 can be used to help teens make healthful food choices. During growth spurts—when teens can grow several inches over a period of a few months—calorie and nutrient needs are much higher than usual. Growth spurts are accompanied by increased appetite, and it's important to make sure your teen is consuming plenty of foods that provide protein and calcium.

Since teens will choose many of their own meals and snacks, it's a good idea to have plenty of healthful foods available that can be quickly prepared or carried in a backpack. Some ideas that are likely to have teenager-appeal:

Dried fruits
Trail mix
Popcorn
Frozen vegan pizza slices
Hummus on pita bread
Calcium-fortified juice or soymilk in individual serving cartons
Bagels
English muffins with almond butter
Burritos
Veggie burgers
Instant soups

Instant hot cereals

Ready-to-eat cereals

Smoothies with frozen fruit, soft tofu, and fortified soymilk

It's critical that teenagers regularly consume high-calcium foods like fortified soymilk and orange juice or calcium-set tofu. You should also include beans, a good source of iron, in foods that teenagers tend to enjoy, such as baked beans, salads with chickpeas, hummus, and burritos.

The widely varying nutrient and calorie needs of the teen years make it difficult to come up with a sample menu for this age group. The menu on page 162 provides approximately 3,000 calories and offers ideas for teen-friendly meals that are packed with good nutrition.

Eating Disorders

While some research suggests that eating disorders are more common among vegetarian teens, this is because girls sometimes adopt a vegetarian or vegan diet as a way to manage and disguise their unhealthy food behavior.[5] That is, the eating disorder comes first and a vegan diet is merely one of many tools aimed at controlling calorie intake. But healthy girls who become vegan or are raised in vegan households are no more likely than anyone else to develop an eating disorder. A vegan diet is not a sign of an eating disorder.

The causes of eating disorders are complex and poorly understood. Parents who are concerned that their child might be adopting unhealthy attitudes toward food should look for these classic signs of eating disorders:

- Unnecessary weight loss that continues beyond three months.
- Meal skipping.
- Avoidance of all foods that appear to be high in calories or that contain fat, such as tofu, meat substitutes, peanut butter, breads, and pastas.

- Compulsive counting of fat grams and calories.
- Offering repeated excuses for not eating.
- Frequent weight checks.
- Complaints about feeling bloated after eating normal portions.
- Ritualistic behavior around food, such as cutting food into tiny pieces or eating only one food at a time.
- Avoiding social situations that involve food.
- Excessive exercise.
- Distorted body image.

REAL VEGAN CHILDREN

Most parents worry at some time or another about their child's diet and nutrient intake. In today's world, where children are bombarded with advertisements for fast foods and have constant access to fatty, salty, sugary, processed foods in school and out, there is a deepening crisis regarding children's nutrition. The evidence lies in the dramatic increases in obesity and diabetes among young Americans over the past several decades.

Questions about meeting nutrient needs on a vegan diet seem to pale in comparison to those larger public health concerns. When it comes to feeding vegan children, parents need to give extra attention to vitamin B_{12}, calcium, vitamin D, and essential fats. Like adults, vegan kids need a reliable source of iodine and plenty of foods that are rich in iron, zinc, and protein. But once your family is in the swing of planning balanced vegan meals, you'll see that it isn't difficult. And we know for a fact that vegan children can thrive.

If you met Ellen, Ciera, Tyler, Will, and Maya, you wouldn't worry about whether children can be vegan—and healthy. These—and other "real vegan children"—are featured on the VeganHealth.org website, and they are proof that kids grow and thrive on diets free of all animal foods.

Sixteen-year-old Ellen is the daughter of Matt Ball, co-founder of Vegan Outreach, and his wife, Anne Green. Ellen has never tasted meat, dairy, or eggs, and she says that food has never been a problem. Her favorite foods? "I love most fake meats, especially fake chicken. In particular, we get fake drumsticks from a local restaurant that are absolutely delicious. I like my dad's cooking as well—homemade bread and pizza, 'French fries,' and baked carrots, pancakes and tofu scramble. And he makes the best chocolate peanut-butter pie. For everyday stuff, I love pasta. I'm also really fond of dried blueberries—they're my favorite snack."

Ellen's mother says that Ellen takes a multivitamin with iron and often takes flaxseed oil and a calcium/vitamin D supplement. She takes a sublingual vitamin B_{12} supplement twice a week.

And there is no doubt that Ellen is thriving on her vegan diet. She takes honor and AP classes, gets straight A's at a top high school, and has an IQ over 140 (higher than either of her parents). In her sophomore year, Ellen scored a perfect 800 on the SAT Math II subject test and a perfect 5 on the AP European History test. And Ellen isn't just smart—she's also an athlete who scored four varsity letters in her first two years of high school (cross-country and track), running on two regional championship cross-country teams and the 2009 regional championship four by 800-meter relay team.

Ellen admits that there were social challenges associated with being vegan in elementary and middle school. "Some kids were rude about it, talking about all the meat they ate and the deer they shot last weekend, but high school has been much, much better. I've met quite a few vegetarians, and a lot more people are sympathetic and curious."

Tyler, Will, and Maya (ages nine, seven, and three), whose parents, Lesley and Ray Parker-Rollins, have raised them in a vegan household, are living examples of happy, healthy vegan children. Says their mom, "I love that our children do not believe that animals are here for our use, and I think their beliefs rub off on other people even when they don't realize it. I also make sure that my children know that they can come to me with any questions, concerns, or ideas they may have regarding their experience living vegan in a non-vegan world."

Lesley frequently downloads information on nutrition from Vegan Outreach, the Physicians Committee for Responsible Medicine, and Dr. Michael Greger to give to skeptical doctors, teachers, coaches, grandparents, and friends. "This way, they know I am making informed choices for my children, and it will educate them on the benefits of a vegan diet at the same time."

Lesley says that her freezer is always stocked with vegan cupcakes and cookies for the many birthday parties that come up in the classroom or at someone's home. Her children also have a shelf of vegan snacks at school to enjoy during snack time. They also enjoy veganized versions of some of the kid-friendly staples like chicken nuggets, macaroni and cheese, pizza, and burgers.

"I wish I could say that their favorite foods were lentil loaf, kale soup, and butternut squash, but they aren't. However, they will eat these or anything else that is put in front of them since they want to get dessert!" Lesley says that all three kids love their dad's pancakes and waffles for breakfast, and like most children, they enjoy pizza and sweets. Other favorites are peanut butter and jelly sandwiches, fruit, raw vegetables, Clif bars, and soy yogurt.

To help Tyler, Will, and Maya understand why their family has chosen a vegan diet, their parents take them for frequent visits to farm animal sanctuaries and events sponsored by Vegan Outreach. Says Lesley, "I do believe our children will be grateful to us one day for teaching them to make compassionate choices for themselves, the animals, and the planet."

Heather and Damian Leughmyer didn't listen to people who insisted that a vegan pregnancy wasn't a good choice. And they proved them wrong when Heather gave birth to a healthy baby girl named Ciera on January 10, 2008.

During her pregnancy, Heather ate a variety of whole grains, vegetables, fruits, legumes, and fortified cereals; she drank fortified juices and soymilk; and took a vegan prenatal vitamin supplement.

Ciera grew and thrived on breast milk, which was supplemented starting at six months with pureed vegetables and then fruits. At almost three years old, Ciera is a healthy, energetic redhead who loves vegan cupcakes, chocolate soy pudding, and spinach. "Yes, she loves spinach," says Heather. "It often surprises people to see someone her age eating so much of a food kids are known to hate, and love every bite. In fact, she likes a variety of vegetables and other foods that many kids won't touch." Heather notes that, as a vegan, Ciera has already been introduced to many foods that some adults have yet to try.

Although Ciera is still too young to comprehend why she is vegan, she adores animals. Heather notes that she will never have to lie to Ciera about where her food comes from. "She will never have to come to the painful realization that she is eating a living, feeling being. Her health is not the only thing benefiting from veganism. Her heart is too."

We invite you to visit the VeganHealth website, where you can see photos of more real vegan children and hear their stories (www.vegan health.org/articles/realveganchildren).

Children and teens can use the food guide in Chapter 7 with the following modifications to the number of servings. Precise servings will vary, though, depending on an individual child's rate of growth and physical activity, so these numbers are meant as general guidelines.

MEAL PLANNING GUIDELINES FOR PRESCHOOLERS, SCHOOL-AGE CHILDREN, AND TEENS		
Food group	Servings	
	4 to 8 years old	Preteens and Teens
Grains	6–8	8–10
Protein-rich foods: Legumes, nuts, and soyfoods	5	6
Vegetables	4	4
Fruits	2–5	2–5
Fats	2	3
Calcium-rich foods	6	10

In addition to foods from the food guide, the following supplements can help your child meet nutrient needs.

Age	B_{12} in daily dose(μg)	B_{12} in two doses per week(μg)*	Iodine (μg)^p	Vitamin D**	DHA
SUPPLEMENTS FOR PRESCHOOLERS, SCHOOL-AGE CHILDREN, AND TEENS					
1–3 years	10–40	375	90	600	200
4–8 years	13–50	500	90	600	200
9–13 years	20–75	750	120	600–1,000	200
14–20 years	25–100	1,000	150	600–1,000	200

*If supplements are taken twice a week rather than daily, use these amounts for each of the two doses.
**Current recommended vitamin D intake is 600 IUs for children over the age of one year. We've provided a range of intakes up to 1,000 IUs per day, since some experts believe higher intakes are beneficial.

A NOTE ABOUT DHA

There are no studies measuring levels of the long-chain omega-3 fats EPA or DHA in vegetarian or vegan children. However, we do know that many healthy children have been raised on vegan diets without supplements of either the long-chain omega-3 fats or the essential fatty acid alpha-linolenic acid (ALA). It's possible that children who are vegan from birth are more efficient at manufacturing DHA and EPA. But until we know more, we recommend a DHA supplement of 100 to 200 milligrams per day for children.

Sample Menu for Preschooler/Kindergarten-Age

BREAKFAST
- ½ cup oatmeal
- ½ cup calcium-fortified orange juice
- 1 slice whole-wheat toast with 1 tablespoon almond butter

SNACK
- ½ cup fortified soymilk
- 1 small carrot muffin

LUNCH
Missing Egg Salad Sandwich

- Small whole-wheat pita pocket
- ½ cup mashed tofu
- ½ tablespoon vegan mayonnaise
- shredded zucchini

- ½ cup calcium-fortified orange juice

SNACK
Fruit smoothie

- ½ frozen banana
- ½ cup strawberries

DINNER
Rice pilaf

- ½ cup brown rice
- ¼ cup lentils
- 2 tablespoons raisins

- ½ cup steamed kale with 1 tablespoon sliced almonds
- ¼ cup vegan ice cream

SNACK
- ½ cup fortified soymilk
- ½ low-fat granola bar

Sample Menu for Twelve-year-old

BREAKFAST
- 2 whole-wheat pancakes cooked in 2 teaspoons margarine
- 1 cup blueberries
- ½ cup fortified soymilk

SNACK
- 5 figs

LUNCH

No Tuna Sandwich

- 2 slices whole-wheat bread
- ½ mashed chickpeas with chopped celery and 1 tablespoon vegan mayonnaise

- Sliced tomatoes
- 1 cup calcium-fortified orange juice

SNACK
- 1 whole-wheat English muffin
- ½ cup tofu-carrot spread (¼ cup soft tofu and ¼ cup cooked carrots)
- 1 cup fortified soymilk

DINNER
- 1 cup brown rice
- 1 cup steamed broccoli
- ½ cup steamed carrots
- ¼ cup peanut sauce

Sample 3,000-calorie Menu for Teenager

BREAKFAST ON THE GO

Protein-rich smoothie

- 1 cup silken tofu
- 1 cup calcium-fortified orange juice
- 1 frozen banana

- English muffin with 2 tablespoons peanut butter

SNACK

- ¼ cup trail mix

LUNCH

Vegan sub sandwich

- 6-inch whole-wheat sub roll
- 4 vegan deli slices
- 2 slices vegan cheese
- Lettuce, tomato, and pickles
- 1 tablespoon vegan mayonnaise

- 1 cup fortified almond milk
- Apple

SNACK

- 2 oatmeal cookies
- 1 cup fortified soymilk

DINNER

Burritos

- 3 medium whole-wheat tortillas
- 1 cup refried beans
- ½ cup mashed avocado
- Chopped tomato and lettuce
- Salsa

- 1 cup brown rice
- 2 cups steamed kale seasoned with 2 teaspoons sesame oil

SNACK

- 2 cups bran flakes
- 1 cup fortified almond milk

CHAPTER 11

VEGAN DIETS FOR PEOPLE OVER FIFTY

We really don't know very much about the eating habits of older vegans. And that's too bad because nutrient needs change with aging in ways that might have particular relevance for those who eat plant-based diets.

The biggest issue for everyone, vegan or not, is that calorie needs for older adults decrease while nutrient needs stay generally the same or—in the cases of calcium, vitamin D, vitamin B_6, and possibly protein—go up. Research shows that some older omnivores and lacto-ovo vegetarians fall short on nutrient intake. We suspect that this is true for some vegans as well.

It's difficult to talk about nutrient needs of people "over fifty" because this is such a diverse group. Meal-planning issues and nutrient needs are likely to change considerably between the ages of fifty-five and eighty-five. For example, while women tend to find that menopause is accompanied by unwanted weight gain, for people in their eighties, getting enough calories can become the challenge. This chapter looks at issues that may affect people at different stages of the later years.

CHANGES IN NUTRIENT NEEDS WITH AGING

The chart on page 167 shows changes in the RDAs for people over fifty. A nutrient of particular concern for all older people is vitamin

B_{12}. There is evidence that some signs of aging—such as loss of hearing, forgetfulness, confusion, and depression—could be related at least in part to inadequate vitamin B_{12} since this vitamin affects the nervous system. A marginal intake of vitamin B_{12} can also raise the risk for stroke, a problem in older people.

This is where vegans might have the edge, as we discussed in Chapter 3. Absorption of vitamin B_{12} from meat, dairy, and eggs declines among a large percentage of older people because of digestive changes. Changes causing decreased absorption may affect as many as 30 percent of people over the age of fifty and 37 percent of those over the age of eighty.[1] However, most of these changes don't affect absorption of vitamin B_{12} from supplements and fortified foods, so health professionals advise all people over the age of 50 to get at least half of their B_{12} from these sources. Many people, though, aren't aware of this recommendation. That's where the vegan advantage comes in, because vegans who are educated about good nutrition are *already* taking B_{12} supplements.

Vitamin D needs are higher for those over the age of seventy. One reason for the increased requirements is that the synthesis of vitamin D from sun exposure declines with aging. In addition, calcium absorption becomes less efficient. While there is much debate about how much calcium people need at all stages of life, adequate vitamin D and calcium are both important for preventing osteoporosis in later years. The current calcium recommendation for those over age fifty is 1,200 milligrams per day, but studies suggest that amounts quite a bit higher are useful in preventing bone loss.[2] It's possible that for all older adults—vegan or not—supplements are necessary to achieve optimal calcium intake.

There has been quite a bit of discussion about protein needs as people age. Lower calorie intake results in slightly higher protein needs, and there is also evidence that protein is utilized less efficiently with aging. The FNB does not recommend an increase in protein intake for older people, but some experts suggest that protein needs could be as much as 25 to 50 percent higher for older people compared to younger adults.[3] Since vegans probably have somewhat higher protein requirements than omnivores, it's important for older people to emphasize protein-rich foods in meals. High protein intakes along with resistance exercise, such as weight-lifting, have been shown to slow the loss of muscle mass that commonly occurs as we age.[4] And protein supplements may improve bone health in older people.

Finally, the RDA for vitamin B_6 is higher for older adults. This shouldn't be a problem for vegans as long as their diets include a variety of whole plant foods.

One other change actually makes diet planning a little easier for older women. After menopause, iron requirements drop by roughly one-half since women no longer lose iron through monthly periods.

The challenges in planning healthy meals for older people aren't all related to changes in nutrient needs. Taste sensitivity declines with aging due to either a decline in the sense of smell or an actual reduction in the number of taste buds. It is a real phenomenon and can lead to over-salting of food or poor appetite. It's hard to eat if food doesn't taste good.

Changes in living situations can have a significant effect on food choices too. Older people who find themselves living alone may find that their interest in cooking and eating suffers. While most neighborhoods offer communal or home-delivered meals for seniors, they are rarely suitable for vegans. Chapter 8 lists options for simplified and convenient meals that can be especially helpful for anyone who is cooking for one.

TIPS FOR OLDER VEGANS

- Watch your calories. As calorie needs begin to decrease with aging, it's important either to cut back on energy intake or—a better idea for all-around health—to increase physical activity.
- Limit empty-calorie junk foods. This is good advice for everyone, but if you are cutting back on calories to manage your

weight, it's important to get the most you can from the foods you are eating. Choose plenty of whole plant foods and fortified foods to meet nutrient needs.

- Eat plenty of vitamin B_6-rich foods like bran flakes, potatoes, tomato juice, bananas, figs, chickpeas, and veggie meats made from soy.
- Take a vitamin D supplement. It's unlikely that older people—vegan or omnivore—can meet needs otherwise.
- Choose plenty of calcium-rich foods, aiming for at least eight servings per day from the Vegan Food Guide. If your diet regularly falls short of calcium, taking a supplement is a good idea.
- It goes without saying that no matter how old you are, a vitamin B_{12} supplement (chewable or sublingual) or plenty of B_{12}-fortified foods is a must for vegans.
- Give your diet a protein boost by consuming plenty of legumes, nut butters, and soy products. Choose quinoa instead of rice or barley because it is one of the most protein-rich grains.
- Seek out condiments and spices that add flavor without excess salt. If you like spicy foods, perk up meals with salsa or cayenne pepper, or add curry powder to beans.
- Don't forget to drink plenty of water. Many older people don't get enough liquids.

THE BUDGET-MINDED VEGAN

If, like many older people, you live on a fixed income, cutting food costs may be a priority. Some of the best vegan nutritional buys include potatoes, dried beans, frozen vegetables (which are just as nutritious as fresh), peanut butter, brown rice, and oatmeal. Refined grains are often cheaper than whole grains, and, if your budget is tight, there is nothing wrong with the occasional serving of regular pasta or white rice. You'll find more tips for planning a healthy vegan diet on a budget in Chapter 8. The menu on page 169 makes use of lower-cost and easy-to-prepare foods.

CHANGES IN NUTRIENT NEEDS WITH AGING

	Age 31–50		Age 51–70		Age 70-plus	
	M	F	M	F	M	F
Calcium AI Milligrams	1,000	1,000	1,200	1,200	1,200	1,200
Vitamin D AI IU	600	600	600	600	800	800
Chromium AI Micrograms	35	25	30	20	30	20
Iron RDA Milligrams	8	18	8	8	8	8
Iron RDA Milligrams Vegetarians	14	33	14	14	14	14
Vitamin B_6 RDA Milligrams	1.3	1.3	1.7	1.5	1.7	1.5
Vitamin B_{12} RDA Micrograms	2.4	2.4	2.4	2.4	2.4	2.4

PROTECTING COGNITIVE FUNCTION

Nutrition plays a role in all aspects of health as people age and that includes cognitive function. We don't have any information about cognitive function in older vegans, but among Seventh-day Adventists, people who eat meat were more than twice as likely to develop dementia.[5]

Cognitive decline may be due, in part, to the production of free radicals, which are normal products of metabolism. Antioxidants, including nutrients like vitamin C and beta-carotene, as well as other plant chemicals, help neutralize free radicals and could support cognitive function. People who adopt vegan diets may have better antioxidant status according to some research.[6]

Higher levels of homocysteine might raise the risk for cognitive decline, which means it is important to get plenty of vitamin B_{12} as well as vitamin B_6 and folate. Although the role of omega-3 fats in protecting cognitive health is controversial, we recommend that vegans over the age of sixty take a daily algae-derived supplement that provides 200 to 300 micrograms of DHA.

Non-dietary factors also play a significant role in keeping the brain young. Exercise seems to be especially important, as is challenging your brain as much as possible by reading, doing crossword puzzles, or learning new skills.

Tips for protecting cognitive function:

- Yes, we sound like a broken record when it comes to this, but we can't say it too often: Make sure you have a reliable source of vitamin B_{12} in your diet.
- Eat an antioxidant-rich diet by consuming lots of fruits and vegetables.
- Take a daily DHA supplement of 200 to 300 micrograms.
- Exercise your body with daily walking, weight training, or an exercise class.
- Exercise your mind: Do crossword puzzles or Sudoku, learn to play bridge, or master a new language.

This sample menu for older people maximizes nutrient intake with affordable, easy-to-prepare meals.

BREAKFAST
- ▸ 1 cup bran flakes
- ▸ ½ cup fortified soymilk
- ▸ 1 banana, sliced

SNACK
- ▸ ½ whole-wheat English muffin
- ▸ 1 tablespoon peanut butter
- ▸ ½ cup grapes

LUNCH
- ▸ 1 cup homemade or reduced-sodium canned black bean soup topped with chopped avocado and tomato
- ▸ Sliced tomatoes
- ▸ 1 slice whole-wheat bread with 1 teaspoon margarine

SNACK
- ▸ 2 graham crackers
- ▸ 1 cup calcium-fortified orange juice

DINNER
- ▸ 1 small baked potato
- ▸ ½ cup baked tofu
- ▸ 1 cup steamed fresh or frozen collards
- ▸ Green salad dressed with vinaigrette
- ▸ ½ cup vegan ice cream

CHAPTER 12

PLANT FOOD ADVANTAGES
Health Benefits of a Vegan Diet

Several decades ago, most research on plant-based diets focused on nutrition problems associated with this "alternative" way of eating. That has changed in the past twenty years or so; now there is a significant focus on the health advantages of eliminating animal foods from menus.

Here is a quick summary of the benefits of plant-based diets:

- Plant foods provide phytochemicals. These are compounds found only in plants, some of which may reduce the risk of heart disease, cancer, and other diseases.
- Plant foods contain fiber, which is associated with a lower risk for cancer, heart disease, and obesity. Animal foods contain no fiber, and people who follow a typical American diet based on meat and dairy generally don't get as much fiber as experts recommend.
- Plant foods contain no cholesterol. Even lean meats like shrimp and white chicken meat are high in cholesterol, and of course, dairy and eggs are loaded with it.
- Plant foods are low in saturated fat. Most of the saturated fat in American diets comes from meat and dairy foods. Replacing saturated fat with unsaturated fat or complex carbohydrates helps reduce blood-cholesterol levels.
- Some plant foods, like olives and nuts, are high in total fat, but they typically contain healthful types of fat.

- Plant foods are excellent sources of nutrients, such as folate, potassium, and vitamins C and E, all of which may be related to lower risks for chronic disease.

The research on diet and chronic disease is complex and conflicting, though, and trying to find solid proof for the benefits of vegetarian diets—and especially vegan diets—hasn't been as easy as you might expect.

RESEARCH ON
VEGETARIANS AND VEGANS

Much of the available information about the health effects of vegetarian diets comes from just a few large epidemiologic studies. (These studies are expensive, so there aren't very many of them.)

- The European Prospective Investigation into Cancer and Nutrition-Oxford (EPIC-Oxford) in the United Kingdom has 65,429 participants including a fairly high number of vegetarians.
- A study of Seventh-day Adventists, the AHS-2, started in 2002 and had 96,194 participants as of 2007. It includes subjects from all fifty states and Canada and has provided preliminary findings based on questionnaires filled out by participants. Seventh-day Adventists are the only group of vegetarians or vegans from the United States whose disease rates have been studied. The Adventist church promotes a vegetarian diet to its members, and 38 percent of the AHS-2 study participants follow a vegetarian diet. Because Adventists also have low rates of smoking and drinking, they are a good population in which to compare vegetarians with meat-eaters.
- We also have findings from an analysis of five other studies that includes vegetarians from the United Kingdom, the United States, and Germany.

HEART DISEASE

People who eat plant-based diets consume less saturated fat and cholesterol and more of the compounds that protect against heart disease. One analysis of five large studies showed that the risk of dying from heart disease was 24 percent lower for vegetarians compared with meat-eaters.[1]

In addition, a number of studies have shown that adopting a vegetarian diet lowers blood cholesterol and the rate of heart disease (we'll look at this more closely in Chapter 13). There is good evidence that vegetarians have lower blood-cholesterol levels than meat-eaters and that vegans have the lowest blood-cholesterol levels of all.

The table below compares cholesterol levels in vegans, omnivores, lacto-ovo vegetarians, and people who eat fish but no other types of meat to desirable levels recommended by the U.S. government's National Cholesterol Education Program.

AVERAGE CHOLESTEROL AND TRIGLYCERIDE LEVELS*

	Desirable levels	Vegans	Lacto-ovo vegetarians	Pesco-vegetarians (they eat fish but no other meat)	Omnivores
Total cholesterol	Less than 200 mg	160	185	196	201
LDL-cholesterol	Less than 100 mg	90.3	106	114	121
HDL-cholesterol	Above 60 mg	52	57	61	55
Ratio of total cholesterol to HDL-cholesterol	Below 3.5:1**	3.1	3.3	3.2	3.7
Triglycerides	Below 150 mg	86	108		107

*Average lipid levels from 17 studies of Western populations between 1980 and 2003. This chart averages blood cholesterol and triglyceride levels from seventeen studies of western populations between 1980 and 2003.[2]

**Your total cholesterol should be no more than 3.5 times higher than your HDL-cholesterol.

The levels of LDL-cholesterol and HDL-cholesterol matter more than total cholesterol. LDL is the so-called "bad" cholesterol that is associated with a higher risk of heart disease. HDL-cholesterol is the "good" or protective form of cholesterol. The ratio of total cholesterol to HDL cholesterol is the best indicator of risk; the lower the ratio, the better.

Total cholesterol in vegans tends to be well below the upper limit of 200 milligrams, and vegans also have low LDL-cholesterol levels. Although they have lower levels of protective HDL-cholesterol, their ratio of total to HDL-cholesterol is better than that of lacto-ovo vegetarians, fish eaters, and meat-eaters. Vegans also have lower triglycerides, a type of fat that is linked to higher risk for heart disease.

HYPERTENSION

Interest in the blood pressure–lowering effect of a vegetarian diet dates back to the early part of the twentieth century. In 1926, one researcher reported that the blood pressure of vegetarian college students increased within two weeks of adding meat to their diets.[3] More recent studies of Seventh-day Adventists show that vegetarians have lower blood pressures and also lower rates of hypertension than omnivores.[4] Some data indicate that vegans have lower blood pressures than lacto-ovo vegetarians. In one British study, meat-eaters were 2½ times as likely as vegans to suffer from hypertension.[5]

The reasons why vegan diets could help lower blood pressure aren't completely understood. Lower body weight and sodium intake account for some but not all of the difference. Diets high in fruits and vegetables are associated with lower blood pressures, and that may be part of the explanation for the protective effects of plant-based diets. Most experts believe that it is a combination of multiple factors that explains the protective effects of plant-based diets.

BODY WEIGHT

Scientists assess body weight by looking at the body mass index (BMI), which is a measure of weight based on height. It's not a perfect assessment, however, because it doesn't account for muscle mass (which weighs more than fat), but it is a helpful tool for comparing populations.

A BMI of 20 to 25 is considered healthy. Above 25 is overweight and over 30 is considered obese. The two tables below display findings from Seventh-day Adventists and British vegetarians. You can see that in both groups, vegans have lower BMIs than people following either lacto-ovo or semi-vegetarian diets.

BODY MASS INDEXES OF SEVENTH-DAY ADVENTISTS[6]

Vegans	Lacto-ovo vegetarians	Pesco-vegetarians (they eat fish but no other meat)	Semi-vegetarians	Meat-eaters
23.6	25.7	26.3	27.3	28.8

BODY MASS INDEXES OF BRITISH VEGETARIANS (FROM THE EPIC-OXFORD STUDY)[7]

	Vegans	Lacto-ovo vegetarians	Pesco-vegetarians	Meat-eaters
Men	22.5	23.4	23.4	24.4
Women	22	22.7	22.7	23.5

OTHER CHRONIC DISEASE CONDITIONS

The preliminary data from the newest study of Adventists shows that vegans were less than half as likely to have diabetes when compared with meat-eaters. While being overweight raises the risk for diabetes, the lower BMI of vegans in this study was determined not to be the only reason for their lower diabetes risk.

Research suggests that vegetarians are less likely to form either renal stones or gallstones, and as we would expect from their higher fiber intake, vegetarians are only about half as likely as omnivores to develop intestinal problems like diverticular disease. Among Seventh-day Adventists, vegetarians are also less likely to develop dementia. So far, we don't have any information about the effects of a vegan diet on these conditions.

VEGETARIAN DIETS AND CANCER

The relationship of diet to cancer has proven to be extremely difficult to study. It's a complex disease and there aren't many markers for cancer risk. That is, we can measure the effects of diet on blood-cholesterol levels and make predictions about how that will affect heart disease risk. But we don't have many blood parameters related to cancer risk that are as straightforward.

There is evidence that how people eat in childhood is linked to their risk later on for developing cancer, which means that it is hard to uncover the links between diet and cancer risk without studying lifelong eating habits And because cancer is such a complex disease, it's possible that the disease process is affected by interactions among different food components and by food components that aren't well-understood. As a result, we have a very poor grasp of what type of diet protects against cancer. A few studies have found that vegetarians have lower cancer rates compared to omnivores, but most haven't shown any difference between the two groups.

The environment of the colon in vegetarians—including the levels of different bacteria and enzymes—differs from meat-eaters in ways that appear to be protective against colon cancer. This is due in part to a higher intake of fiber, which is linked to a lower risk for cancer. Vegetarians and vegans also eat more fruits and vegetables and have a higher intake of antioxidants than omnivores. But while it's generally believed that this lowers cancer risk, the evidence has weakened over the past few years as some recent studies haven't supported a link between fruit and vegetable intake and cancer. Soyfoods are linked to reduced risk for both breast and prostate cancer although this, too, is an area that needs more study.

In contrast to the possible protective effects of plant foods, certain animal foods may raise cancer risk. Red and processed meats are linked to a higher risk for colon, stomach, and possibly bladder cancer. Some researchers believe that eliminating meat from the diet is more beneficial for reducing colon cancer than eating more fiber. Others suggest that eating meat in adolescence raises the risk for breast cancer later in life. There is also evidence to suggest that high dairy consumption raises the risk for prostate cancer.

Based on these findings, it would seem that vegans should have a lower risk for cancer, but we don't have enough research to draw any conclusions. And because of conflicting findings, we haven't yet been able to define the diet that protects against cancer. Cancer experts advise

 ## What about the China Study?

Some readers may wonder why we didn't cite findings from the China Study in this chapter. The China Study compared the types of food consumed and average disease rates in different counties in China, mostly during the 1980s. The results showed that the more plant products and less animal products consumed in a given county, the lower the rates of most chronic diseases, such as heart disease and many cancers. The China Study was an ecological study, which you may recall from Chapter 2 is a study that compares population groups rather than individuals. Ecological studies can add to our understanding about diet and health, and often give rise to hypotheses that stimulate further research, but they carry less weight than other types of epidemiologic studies.

Additionally, most of the participants in the China Study were neither vegetarian nor vegan, making it difficult to draw specific conclusions about the health benefits of these diets. This is not a criticism of the China Study. It is just to say that it doesn't provide information for our purpose in this chapter, which is to describe research on the health of vegans.

eating a diet rich in fruits and vegetables, fiber, and phytochemicals from plant foods, while minimizing fat from animal foods. Consequently, it seems like vegans have advantages that may lower their cancer risk.

DISEASE RISK IN VEGANS

Because vegans make up such a small percentage of the population, findings about their disease rates are few. What little data we have suggests that vegans have a lower body weight, lower blood-cholesterol levels, and lower blood pressures, all of which may offer significant protection against chronic disease. But one study also suggested that vegans have a higher rate of bone fracture than meat-eaters, although this occurred only when their calcium intake is low.

These findings may not be very exciting and they may surprise you. But while they aren't necessarily what we want to see—it's *all the research there is*! What we know about typical vegan diets and vegan health parameters tells us that vegans should have a lower risk for many chronic diseases. And that may very well be the case, but we simply don't have the studies yet to prove it.

However, we do know that choosing more plant foods and fewer animal foods is important for overall health and disease prevention. For those who are making lifestyle changes to manage chronic disease, a vegan diet can be helpful, as we'll see in the next chapter.

CHAPTER 13

MANAGING WEIGHT, HEART DISEASE, AND DIABETES

We've seen that vegans have lower cholesterol levels, less hypertension and diabetes, and a lower rate of obesity than meat-eaters. So it seems logical that a vegan diet is good therapy for the chronic conditions that are all too common among Americans today. And the research suggests that this may very well be the case—that going vegan can be a smart approach to managing high cholesterol, diabetes, and high blood pressure. To put these benefits to work for you and your family, it helps to know just which aspects of a vegan diet are most beneficial.

BENEFITS OF VEGAN DIETS FOR MANAGING CARDIOVASCULAR DISEASE

Cardiovascular disease (CVD) refers to conditions that involve narrowed or blocked blood vessels, raising risk for heart attack and stroke. CVD is sometimes used interchangeably with the term "heart disease."

There has been much discussion of late in the media and among research experts challenging the long-held belief that saturated fats raise the risk for heart disease.[1,2] Extensive analyses have shown that replacing saturated fat in the diet with refined carbohydrates doesn't lower heart disease risk; it increases it. This has led to the suggestion that the real problem is refined carbohydrates, not saturated fat.

Actually, the problem is probably both refined carbohydrates and saturated fat. We know from a large body of research that replacing saturated fat with healthier fats—poly- and monounsaturated ones— reduces blood-cholesterol levels and is associated with a lower risk for heart disease.[3] Similar benefits occur when saturated fat is replaced with carbohydrates from whole, unrefined plant foods. It's not a matter of giving up carbs or fats; it's a matter of choosing the right ones.

In theory, you could eat a high saturated fat diet by loading up on coconut and palm oil, but the reality is that switching to a diet based on plant foods is pretty much guaranteed to substantially lower your saturated fat intake. Vegans eat much less saturated fat than meat-eaters and, as we saw in Chapter 12, they have lower levels of total blood cholesterol and, more importantly, of LDL-cholesterol. This is the "bad" cholesterol that is responsible for increased deposits of plaque in the arteries, which causes them to narrow and even become blocked. Narrowed arteries also cause an increase in blood pressure, and high blood pressure in turn can damage arteries—a vicious and potentially life-threatening cycle.

In addition to their lower saturated fat intake, vegans enjoy other advantages thanks to their diet:

- Plant foods are high in antioxidants, which may prevent cholesterol deposits from forming in the arteries, although not all research supports this theory.
- Vegans tend to have lower blood pressure, putting them at a reduced risk for a heart attack or stroke.
- Vegans are likely to eat more soyfoods than omnivores, and there is evidence suggesting that compounds in soy help make blood vessels more elastic—a factor that reduces the risk for atherosclerosis. Soy protein may also lower blood-cholesterol levels. (More on this in Chapter 15.)
- Nuts, which often play an important role in vegan diets, are linked to a reduced risk for heart disease.[4]

BENEFITS OF VEGAN DIETS FOR
CONTROLLING TYPE-2 DIABETES

Type-1 diabetes is an autoimmune disorder in which the pancreas doesn't produce enough (or any) insulin. Without insulin, blood glucose can't get into cells, and the cells starve. People with this disease require lifelong insulin therapy. But by far the more prevalent type of diabetes is type 2, in which enough insulin is produced, but the cells become resistant to it.

Being overweight and inactive raises the risk for type-2 diabetes. The disease is on the rise not only among Americans but also among people in developing countries because they are adopting American-style eating habits, including more fatty animal foods and refined carbohydrates.

Type-2 diabetes used to be called adult onset diabetes because it occurred primarily in older people, but we are beginning to see it at astounding rates among teens and even children in the United States.

Some people with type-2 diabetes take medication, but the condition can often be managed very well through diet and exercise. Sometimes, losing a few pounds is enough to improve glucose control. There are a number of reasons why a diet based on whole plant foods could be helpful for controlling diabetes:

- A vegan diet doesn't guarantee that you'll be slender, but vegans are less likely to be obese. Weight loss is often the single most effective way to control diabetes.
- Although vegan diets are typically high in carbohydrates, they tend to have a low glycemic index, which could be an advantage in controlling diabetes. The glycemic index is a measure of how quickly carbohydrates are digested and absorbed. We'll discuss this further later in the chapter.
- People with diabetes are at especially high risk for cardiovascular disease. So the factors in plant-based diets that reduce risk for CVD can be especially important for those with diabetes.

- The lower rates of hypertension in vegans can be important, too, in controlling some of the complications of diabetes.

LOW-FAT VEGAN DIETS FOR
TREATING HEART DISEASE AND DIABETES:
THE RESEARCH

Dr. Nathan Pritikin was an early advocate of a vegan diet that limited all fats. His approach was effective in reducing cholesterol, blood sugar, and blood pressure levels.

A few years later and using a similar although not-quite-vegan diet, Dr. Dean Ornish launched a study called the Lifestyle Heart Trial.[5] The subjects were people with moderate to severe coronary heart disease. Some followed the usual diet that was recommended for heart disease and others adopted a comprehensive lifestyle plan which included a 10 percent fat vegetarian diet (consisting almost entirely of whole plant foods with the addition of nonfat dairy), aerobic exercise, stress management, support groups, and smoking cessation.

The subjects who followed a standard cholesterol-lowering plan actually got worse over the course of the study (atherosclerosis increased by nearly 28 percent after five years), but the health of subjects in the lifestyle group improved. Atherosclerosis in this group decreased by nearly 8 percent after five years.

More recently, researchers with the Physicians Committee for Responsible Medicine (PCRM) looked at the effects of a low-fat vegan diet on type-2 diabetes.[6] Subjects in the test group were instructed to follow a low-fat vegan diet based on whole plant foods with no limits on carbohydrates, calories, or portion sizes. Those in the control group followed a typical American Diabetes Association (ADA) diet, which uses portion control and carbohydrate counting and includes animal foods.

With their higher carbohydrate intake, it might seem like those on the low-fat vegan diet would get worse, but they didn't. They lost more weight, even though they didn't count calories or measure their food, and their blood glucose was better controlled.

These effective approaches for reversing heart disease and controlling diabetes have two things in common. First, they are based on whole plant foods rather than refined carbohydrates. And second, they are very low in fat—as low as 10 to 15 percent of calories in some cases.

It's likely that many of the benefits of these diets are explained by weight loss (which reduces blood cholesterol), reduced intake of saturated fat, and perhaps protective compounds in plants. It may be that simply eating a vegan diet—based mostly on whole, unprocessed foods—and reducing calorie intake is enough to achieve therapeutic results. We'll see below that whether or not these diets need to be low in total fat is an issue of much debate.

FAT AND CHRONIC DISEASE

Reducing intake of saturated fat is important for reducing LDL-cholesterol levels, but it's possible that including some higher-fat plant foods in the diet is better for managing disease. In Chapter 12, we talked about the ideal cholesterol profile for reducing heart disease: low LDL-cholesterol and high HDL-cholesterol. When all types of fat in the diet are replaced with mostly carbohydrates, both LDL- and HDL-cholesterol drop.[7] But replacing saturated fat with healthful plant fats lowers LDL-cholesterol without affecting the good HDL-cholesterol. Monounsaturated fat also improves glucose control in people with diabetes when it replaces saturated fat or carbohydrates in the diet.[8]

This has led some researchers to conclude that the healthiest diet is one that is very low in saturated fat but not too low in total fat.[9] The traditional Mediterranean diet is an example of a healthful eating pattern that includes good fats, especially the monounsaturated fats found in nuts, olives, and avocado.

How much this matters for people following vegan diets is still up for debate. But low HDL levels seem to be an important risk factor for women in particular and for those with type-2 diabetes.[10] HDL levels also matter a great deal for people who are overweight and sedentary. For example, in the EPIC-Norfolk study, the ratio of total cholesterol to HDL-cholesterol was more strongly linked to heart disease risk than LDL levels.[11]

Some nutritionists believe that people who cook with olive oil, which is rich in monounsaturated fat, are likely to consume more vegetables (because the olive oil makes them taste so good). So it may be that vegetables are the protective factor and olive oil is just an innocent bystander. But olive oil also contains compounds that affect blood-clotting factors associated with heart disease risk.[12] This suggests that small amounts of olive oil could be beneficial—or at the very least not harmful. While nobody knows exactly how much fat is ideal, it seems clear that a very low-fat diet is not the answer for everyone who needs to reduce disease risk.

Another type of fat in foods—trans fats—should definitely be avoided.[13] Although small amounts of trans fats are found naturally in foods, most comes from processed foods made with partially hydrogenated fats. Hydrogenation is the process that turns vegetable oils into solid fat. Consuming trans fat raises the levels of bad LDL-cholesterol, reduces protective HDL-cholesterol, and is associated with a higher risk of both heart disease and diabetes. The American Heart Association recommends limiting trans fat to 1 percent of total calories. That's such a tiny amount that practically speaking, it means you should just avoid all foods that list "partially hydrogenated" oils on the label. (If the label says "fully hydrogenated" or "hydrogenated," the fats have been turned into saturated, not trans, fats. And it's still a good idea to avoid saturated fats.)

Although the amount of trans fat in a food must be listed on the label by law, if the amount is less than ½ gram, the label can say that the food contains "0" grams of trans fat. Since the upper limit for trans fat intake on an 1,800-calorie diet would be two grams per day, eating foods with small amounts of trans fat can add up quickly.

THE GLYCEMIC INDEX:
HOW CARBOHYDRATES AFFECT DISEASE RISK

Carbohydrates are digested and absorbed into the bloodstream as glucose, sometimes called blood sugar. When glucose levels rise, the hormone insulin is released into the blood. Insulin helps cells absorb fat and glucose from the blood, allowing the cells to use these nutrients for energy. Some carbohydrates are converted to glucose more gradually than others. The glycemic index (GI) is a measure of how quickly carbohydrates are broken down and absorbed into the blood. A meal with a high GI causes a surge in the release of insulin, which is associated with increased risk for CVD, diabetes, and possibly cancer.

Foods with a low GI can help with weight control since they help promote the use of body fat for energy, and they also tend to be more satisfying.[14] Diets that are very high in protein are based on the idea that carbohydrates—because of their effects on insulin—are responsible for weight gain. But vegans are typically closer to their ideal body weight than omnivores, despite their higher carbohydrate intakes. And the PCRM studies showed that people on very high carbohydrate diets lose weight and have better blood-glucose control.

The key is to choose carbohydrate-rich foods with low GIs, which means eating more unprocessed, whole plant foods in place of refined carbohydrates. Most types of processing seem to affect the GI. For example, while beans typically have a low GI, the index tends to rise the longer the beans are cooked. And grinding grains into flour increases the GI. The amount of fiber in a food affects its GI, but other factors, some of them fairly obscure, are even more important.

In fact, sometimes the glycemic index makes no sense. Because the type of starch in a food impacts its GI, pasta made from white flour actually has a lower GI than brown rice.

And the glycemic index doesn't always tell the whole story about the effects of a food on blood glucose. Some foods have a high GI, but they contain so little carbohydrate that it doesn't matter. Carrots are a prime example.

Finally, foods that are high in the simple sugar fructose—including table sugar—have a relatively low GI. But some research suggests that a large amount of fructose in the diet is linked to obesity, heart disease, diabetes, and high blood pressure. When it comes to added sweeteners, a good rule of thumb is to minimize all of them regardless of their GI.

Despite these quirks, it's fairly easy to make healthy food choices to keep the GI low in your meals.

REDUCE THE GLYCEMIC INDEX OF MEALS WITH EASY REPLACEMENTS

Choose these foods . . .	More often than these. . .
Bread made from unground whole, cracked, or sprouted grains (sometimes called "grainy" bread)	Breads made from flour
Sweet potatoes	White potatoes
Whole potatoes cooked in their skin	Mashed potatoes
Spaghetti, oats, and barley	White rice
Rolled oats or muesli	Ready-to-eat or instant cereals
Whole raw fruits	Juice or cooked or dried fruits
Raw or lightly steamed vegetables	Canned or thoroughly cooked vegetables
Regular full-fat soymilk	"Lite" or reduced-fat soymilk
Beans cooked from scratch	Canned beans
Foods flavored with acidic ingredients, such as lemon or lime juice, vinegar, and tomato sauce	Foods flavored with sweet sauces
Nuts and seeds	Snack chips
Meals with small amounts of added fat and high-protein foods like tofu and tempeh	Low-fat, low-protein meals

PUTTING IT ALL TOGETHER:
FOOD CHOICES FOR MANAGING CHRONIC DISEASE

It doesn't matter whether you need to reduce heart disease risk or control diabetes, the guidelines on how to eat are generally the same. For many people, simply losing weight and getting regular exercise is all it takes. Here are some other dietary changes that are important.

- Reduce your saturated fat intake. Vegans are automatically off to a good start in this regard, since most plant foods are naturally low in saturated fat. (The type of saturated fat in coconut oil appears to be less harmful than other types, but all added fats should be used in moderation.)
- Replace some of the saturated fat in your diet with foods that are rich in monounsaturated fats—olive and canola oil, olives, avocadoes, and nuts. These foods help lower LDL-cholesterol without reducing protective HDL-cholesterol.
- Include one to two servings of nuts in your daily menu since they have been shown to reduce LDL-cholesterol and have other heart-healthy factors.
- Avoid trans fats. They are found in any food that lists "partially hydrogenated" vegetable oil or fat on the label. Some brands of vegan cream cheese may contain partially hydrogenated oils.
- Increase your intake of whole, fiber-rich plant foods rather than refined carbohydrates.
- You don't need to eliminate foods with a high GI from your diet, but it may help to emphasize foods with a low glycemic index (refer to the chart on page 186).
- It may be a good idea to include soyfoods in your diet since soy protein has been shown to reduce cholesterol levels.
- Reduce sodium intake if you have hypertension. Not everyone is salt-sensitive, but a diet high in salt is frequently related to high blood pressure, and it can also have a negative impact on bone

health. Getting enough potassium is just as important as reducing sodium intake for managing blood pressure. The best sources of potassium are carrot, orange, and tomato juices, white beans, lentils, sweet potatoes, spinach, Swiss chard, beet greens, sea vegetables, potatoes, dried fruit, and tomato sauce.

- Eat plenty of fruits and vegetables since these foods are high in antioxidants, which appear to protect against a number of diseases.
- Make sure you are meeting the requirements for omega-3 fats as discussed in Chapter 5.
- Talk to your doctor about alcohol. Moderate intake can help raise the good HDL-cholesterol. But for women, even low levels of alcohol consumption can put them at a higher risk for breast cancer.
- Keep in mind that specific needs and recommendations vary depending on your particular health issues. These are general guidelines that can help most people manage CVD and type-2 diabetes, but they may not be right for everyone.

FAT AND WEIGHT CONTROL

Ounce for ounce, fat has twice the calories of protein or carbohydrate. Advocates of very low-fat diets note that the less fat you eat, the fewer calories you are likely to consume and the slimmer you will stay. Some people find that adopting a low-fat diet helps them lose weight without having to count calories or measure food intake. But for long-term weight control, there is evidence that including *some* higher fat foods in menu plans is helpful. When researchers compare weight loss on diets with different levels of fat, some subjects feel that the higher-fat diets are more satisfying.[15] Eating a little bit of fat—usually in the form of nuts or nut butter—can make it easier to stick to a lower-calorie diet over the long-term.

In the Nurses' Health Study, nuts in particular seemed to help prevent weight gain. Over an eight-year period, women who ate nuts two or three times a week gained less weight than those who rarely ate nuts, even when they had similar calorie intakes.[16]

Nuts are unique foods because they are high in protein, fiber, and fat. Their consumption may give a boost to the enhanced metabolism that normally occurs after a meal.[17] And whole nuts are hard to chew completely, which might result in incomplete digestion and fewer calories absorbed. This may help explain why peanut butter doesn't seem to have the same benefits as whole nuts for weight control.

We are not suggesting a free-for-all when it comes to fat intake. It's definitely hard to keep calorie intake low or moderate if you are dousing your food with oil. But including some plant fat, especially monounsaturated fat, in a vegan diet may have advantages for controlling chronic disease and for weight loss compared with eliminating all fats.

PLANNING VEGAN DIETS FOR WEIGHT LOSS

There is no great secret about how to lose weight: Eat less, exercise more. It's hardly surprising that Americans are more overweight than ever since studies of eating habits show that we consume more calories than we did a decade ago. Americans are also less physically active than in times past.

While calories are the real issue in weight loss and gain, where you get those calories may affect your dieting success. Good food choices can help control hunger, making it easier to lose weight and keep the weight off. Use the food guide in Chapter 7 to plan your daily intake. Most people need more than the 1,600 calories provided by the minimum number of servings in the food guide, so add servings from any of the groups to achieve a calorie intake that is comfortable for you and contributes to a slow, steady weight loss. As you make menu choices, keep the following suggestions in mind:

- Find that happy balance between too much and too little fat. Some people have success with weight loss by consuming less fat while others find that including some fat in their meals makes the diet more satisfying and helps with long-term weight control. A good goal is 22 to 27 grams of fat for every 1,000 calories you consume. See Chapter 5 for a quick guide to the amount of fat in different plant foods.

- Get enough protein. There is evidence that protein is better at preventing hunger than either carbohydrate or fat—that is, protein can help you feel satisfied with fewer calories. Boosting protein intake during a weight-loss program can also help preserve muscle tissue so that the body burns more fat and less muscle. Protein-rich plant foods like legumes, soy products, and nuts represent the best of all worlds. They are high in protein but also rich in many protective compounds like fiber and phytochemicals. They also happen to have a low glycemic index.

- Choose foods with a low glycemic index. The easiest way to do this is to concentrate on eating whole, unrefined plant foods. It doesn't mean avoiding all foods that contain carbohydrate.

- Eat lots of vegetables and fresh fruits to fill your stomach with nutrients and fiber without resorting to empty or excess calories.

SAMPLE MENUS

Low GI, Moderate Fat Menu: 1,500 calories

BREAKFAST

Sunny Scrambled Tofu

▸ 1 cup tofu scrambled in 1 teaspoon olive oil with ¼ cup onions, 1 tablespoon nutritional yeast, and 2 tablespoons toasted sunflower seeds

▸ 1 slice "grainy" bread (made from whole grains that haven't been ground into flour)
▸ 1 cup mixed raw fruit

SNACK

Smoothie

▸ ½ frozen banana
▸ ½ cup berries
▸ ½ cup fortified almond milk

LUNCH

▸ 1 ½ cups mushroom-barley soup
   (½ cup cooked barley and ½ cup cooked mushrooms)
▸ 1 slice whole-grain bread with 2 tablespoons almond butter
▸ Tossed green salad with vinaigrette dressing containing 1 teaspoon olive oil

SNACK

▸ ½ cup white bean hummus (made with white beans and sundried tomatoes instead of garbanzos and tahini)
▸ 2 cups raw vegetable strips

DINNER

▸ 2 cups raw vegetable soup made with kale, cucumber, tomatoes, ¼ cup avocado, and seasoned with miso and nutritional yeast
▸ ½ cup cubed baked sweet potato tossed with ½ cup cubed, seasoned tempeh

Low GI, Moderate Fat Menu: 1,800 calories

BREAKFAST

- ▸ 1 cup oatmeal made from steel cut oats, topped with ½ cup chopped figs
- ▸ ½ cup fortified soymilk
- ▸ 1 slice "grainy" bread with 2 tablespoons almond butter

SNACK

- ▸ 1 slice pumpernickel bread with tofu spread (¼ cup soft tofu pureed with 2 tablespoons cooked carrots or other vegetable)

LUNCH

Quinoa salad

- ▸ 1 cup cooked quinoa
- ▸ ½ cup small red beans
- ▸ 1 tablespoon chopped walnuts
- ▸ herbs to taste
- ▸ lemon dressing made with 1 teaspoon olive oil plus lemon juice to taste

- ▸ 1 cup vegetable soup
- ▸ Fresh fruit

SNACK

- ▸ 2 cups raw vegetables
- ▸ ½ cup guacamole (¼ cup avocado and ¼ cup salsa or tomatoes)

DINNER

Bean, pasta, and greens soup

- ▸ ½ cup pasta
- ▸ ½ cup white beans
- ▸ ½ cup cooked kale in vegetable broth

- ▸ 1 cup raw shredded cabbage tossed with 2 tablespoons peanut sauce
- ▸ 1 glass red wine (or replace with small dessert if you prefer)

Special Medical Conditions

Two medical conditions—type-1 diabetes and kidney disease—are beyond the scope of this book. But we want to address them briefly, if only to assure you that people with these conditions can be vegan.

Type-1 Diabetes
As in type-2 diabetes, people with type-1 diabetes may benefit from eating more whole plant foods, which result in a slower release of carbohydrate into the blood. But while we've heard a number of anecdotal reports in support of this theory, there haven't yet been studies to confirm it. Whether or not a plant-based diet has any specific advantages, though, there is no reason to think that those with type-1 diabetes can't be vegan.

If you have type-1 diabetes and want to eat a vegan diet, stick to mostly fiber-rich, whole plant foods and avoid refined grains, added sugars, and sugary drinks. As with any dietary change in type-1 diabetes, you'll want to work closely with your health professional to monitor blood-sugar levels and insulin needs.

Kidney Disease
Plant-based diets have been shown to be beneficial in reducing the markers of kidney disease. This may be due to their lower protein levels, but it could also be from their effect on blood-cholesterol levels and blood pressure and their antioxidant content. People with moderate kidney disease may benefit from a vegan diet—especially one that's free of high-sodium, high-protein vegetarian meats.

Once someone is on dialysis, following a vegan diet becomes more difficult because of the need to restrict potassium and phosphorus, while at the same time insuring adequate protein intake. Planning such a diet is beyond the scope of this book, but we recommend *The Vegetarian Diet for Kidney Disease Treatment* by Joan Brookhyser, a registered dietitian and board-certified specialist in renal nutrition.

While vegetarian meats should be restricted for people with chronic kidney disease, they can play a role in the diet of people on dialysis because they provide high-quality protein. See VeganHealth.org/articles/kidney for a list of vegetarian meats and their saturated fat, potassium, phosphorus, and sodium contents.

CHAPTER 14

SPORTS NUTRITION

There is no question that vegan diets are suitable for competitive sports. Some of the most talented athletes in the world—like ultramarathoner Scott Jurek, world champion boxer Keith Holmes, and professional football star and Heisman Trophy–winner Desmond Howard—have enjoyed successful careers as vegans.

Most of us aren't in their league, of course. If you're hitting the gym two or three times a week to work out, you probably don't need to change a thing about your vegan diet (assuming you're already following our guidelines for healthy eating). It may be that those who train competitively don't need to change much either. Athletes who eat enough to satisfy their appetite will often meet their protein needs without even trying, and they will get a boost in iron intake too. But since vegan diets are typically lower in calories, protein, well-absorbed iron, creatine, and carnitine, it's worth giving these issues some added attention. We'll also discuss carnosine because there has been interest in the relationship of this amino acid to athletic performance.

MEETING ENERGY NEEDS

Exercise efficiency, gender, non-exercise habits, and genetics all affect calorie requirements. And because needs vary with every individual, there is no set formula for determining your energy requirements; it's a matter of experimentation.

For weight lifters, inadequate calorie intake can inhibit muscle growth. Consuming adequate calories preserves muscle protein that would otherwise be used for energy. Pay attention to hunger signals to know whether you are eating enough. For a ballpark figure, one study found that novice male weight lifters lowered body fat while increasing muscle mass and size when they consumed about 18 calories per pound of body weight per day (3,240 calories per day for a 180-pound person).[1] In another study, highly trained male bodybuilders ate 22.7 calories per pound (4,086 calories per day for a 180-pound person).[2]

Teen athletes and others with high calorie needs may find it a challenge to eat enough, but a few simple additions to your diet can help boost calories:

- Include more refined grains in meals. While whole grains are normally the best choice for optimal health, athletes who eat a large quantity of food can afford to eat more processed foods than non-athletes. Because of their lower fiber content, processed foods are less filling. Spaghetti is a good option since its carbohydrate is more slowly released into the bloodstream compared with other processed grains.
- Use moderate amounts of olive oil on salads and for sautéing vegetables.
- Snack on nuts or trail mix, and add avocado to sandwiches to boost fat and calorie intake.
- Add tofu or tempeh to salads or mix it into grain dishes to increase calorie, fat, and protein content of meals.
- Add silken tofu to fruit smoothies.

PROTEIN

Although current government recommendations don't include a separate protein RDA for athletes, opinions about protein needs of athletes vary considerably. And needs may be quite different depending on whether you are engaged in endurance or strength training.

Strength Athletes

Whether the protein needs of strength athletes are any greater than the general population is a subject of debate. There is a legitimate argument for needs ranging anywhere from 0.8 to 1.7 grams of protein per kilogram (0.36 to 0.77 per pound) of healthy body weight. Higher protein intake might be more important for people who are starting a strength routine, and needs might decrease in those who have already fulfilled most of their muscle mass potential.

In a 2009 joint position paper on nutrition and athletic perormance, the American College of Sports Medicine (ACSM), the American Dietetic Association (ADA), and Dietitians of Canada suggested that vegetarian athletes need 1.3 to 1.8 grams of protein per kilogram of body weight, which translates to 0.6 to 0.8 grams per pound.[3]

Here are some practical tips for strength athletes:

- If you are beginning a workout regimen to build muscle mass, make sure to eat plenty of high-protein plant foods, such as legumes or soyfoods. You might consider consuming a protein powder shake providing around 20 grams of protein before or after working out. Once you reach a point where you are not gaining additional muscle mass, this additional dose of protein probably won't be necessary (except for the most serious competitive athletes).
- If you are trying to lose weight, make sure you are eating plenty of protein-rich foods and consider adding a protein powder shake.
- Eating a high-protein food right after working out can increase muscle mass.

Every person is different, so it takes some experimenting to find the right balance. The menu on page 204 is one example of a high-protein diet for athletes.

Endurance Athletes

Endurance athletes may need less protein as they become better trained because, according to the 2009 position paper, protein turnover may become more efficient with training. At the earlier stages of training, you may need as much as 1.2 to 1.4 grams of protein per kilogram of body weight—which translates to 1.3 to 1.55 grams per kilogram for vegan endurance athletes (0.6 to 0.7 grams per pound of body weight).[4]

It can be easier for endurance athletes to meet protein needs simply because they consume more calories. If you are not losing weight and are consuming high-protein foods, you're likely to get plenty of protein. But you might want to calculate your individual needs and track your intake for a few days using the chart on pages 19–20 just to make sure.

When Protein Falls Short

While protein isn't a huge worry for vegan athletes, it's possible to experience muscle damage from a diet that doesn't meet needs. A sixteen-year-old competitive swimmer in Italy who was avoiding almost all high-protein foods suffered temporary, but serious, muscle damage, presumably due to inadequate protein.[5] His muscle damage didn't occur unnoticed; he suffered obvious fatigue and muscle pain. It's a rare and unusual case, but it does illustrate the need to make sure you're eating enough high-protein foods. If you are, and you aren't suffering from muscle pain or unusual fatigue, it's safe to assume that you're getting enough protein.

CARBOHYDRATE AND FAT

Carbohydrates serve as a primary fuel source in distance events, and people who try to cut back on "carbs" often compromise their performance. Vegans are in good standing in this regard, since plant-based diets are typically high in carbohydrates.

According to the ACSM and ADA, low-fat diets—less than 20 percent of calories—are not associated with improved performance. Both groups recommend that athletes consume between 20 and 35 percent of calories from fat. A slightly higher fat intake may be advantageous for trained athletes since they use a higher percentage of fat for energy than non-athletes.

IRON

Iron needs don't increase for strength athletes, but the American College of Sports Medicine recommends that all endurance athletes, especially distance runners, aim for iron intakes that are about 70 percent higher than the RDA.

This raises some questions for vegan endurance athletes. As we talked about in Chapter 6, the RDA for iron is increased by a factor of 1.8 for vegetarians. Like many other nutrition professionals, we believe that this is more iron than most vegetarians and vegans actually need. While some vegan endurance athletes might choose to take a modest daily iron supplement, we hesitate to recommend this since most vegans probably won't need it. However, if you are a menstruating woman involved in endurance sports, you should probably get your iron checked on a regular basis. In fact, the ACSM and ADA recommend that all women athletes be regularly screened to assess their iron status, and screening can be especially important for teen athletes and pregnant women.

PERFORMANCE ENHANCERS

A number of supplements, which include amino acids and other protein-type compounds, are marketed to athletes to enhance their performance.

Creatine

Creatine is the only nutritional supplement that has been consistently shown to improve strength and muscle mass in strength athletes in a large number of clinical trials. It's thought to reduce fatigue during repeated, short bursts of intense exercise—the type that occurs with weight lifting, sprinting, soccer, rugby, and hockey. Less fatigue during sprinting and weight lifting means increased training and greater results.

Humans synthesize creatine in their liver and kidneys, and meat-eaters consume around 1 to 2 grams of creatine per day (although about 30 percent of it is destroyed in cooking). There is no creatine in vegetarian diets, though, and not surprisingly, vegetarians have lower levels of creatine in their blood, urine, red blood cells, and muscle tissue. Some studies have shown that vegetarians benefit more from creatine supplementation than meat-eaters.[6] Fortunately, creatine supplements are vegan.

Creatine supplements are usually taken in two phases for loading and maintenance.

Loading: Take 20 to 30 grams of creatine per day, divided into small doses over the course of the day, for a total of six days.

Maintenance: The usual dose of 2 grams per day is meant for meat-eaters, which means that the dose for vegans may be closer to 2.7 to 3.4 grams per day. Some researchers suggest taking creatine only every other month to maximize its effects. Taking it with a sugar solution, such as a sports drink or fruit juice, increases the rate at which muscles absorb creatine.

According to the ACSM, the most common adverse effects of creatine supplementation are fluid gain, cramping, nausea, and diarrhea. Although its use is widely debated, the ACSM says that it is generally considered safe for adults. That said, there have been anecdotal reports of dehydration, muscle strains or tears, and kidney damage, so it's important to let your health-care professional know if you are taking creatine.

Carnitine

Carnitine (also known as L-carnitine and acetyl-L-carnitine) is an amino acid found in meat and dairy products. It's needed for fat metabolism and is promoted for weight loss and improved performance. According to the ACSM, however, it hasn't been shown to help with either.

While there is very little carnitine in plant foods, it can be synthesized by the liver and kidneys. Vegans, vegetarians, and people who consume lower-fat, high-carbohydrate diets have lower blood levels of carnitine. There is no indication that this is unhealthy, and we don't know if it has any bearing on athletic performance. In one study, vegans who took supplements of 120 milligrams of carnitine per day for two months excreted more carnitine in their urine, but the levels in their plasma didn't increase significantly. This suggests that most of the carnitine was being lost in the urine.[7]

There is no evidence that vegans need to take carnitine, but since non-vegetarians typically eat 100 to 300 milligrams of carnitine per day, it is probably safe for vegans to take supplements providing that amount. Solgar brand carnitine is made by yeast fermentation of beet sugar and is one option available to vegans. If you take carnitine, watch for side effects, including nausea and diarrhea.

Carnosine and Beta-Alanine

Carnosine (also known as beta-alanyl-L-histidine) is a molecule made up of two amino acids, beta-alanine and histidine. Animals, including humans, produce it in various tissues, especially the muscles and the brain. Plant foods don't contain any, and one study has shown that vegetarians have 50 percent less carnosine than meat-eaters in their muscle tissue.[8]

Although the amino acid beta-alanine isn't required in the diet (the body makes its own), beta-alanine supplements have been shown to increase muscle carnosine levels. In fact, only supplements of beta-alanine, not carnosine itself, have been tested on athletic performance in human subjects.

In the ACSM position paper, beta-alanine doesn't appear on the list of performance enhancers "that perform as claimed." But about half a dozen studies have shown that approximately 6 grams of beta-alanine in doses spread over a day, for a period of four or more weeks, results in improved ability to perform, particularly during bouts of cycling. Not all studies have shown a significant benefit, though.

The athletic performance of some individuals might benefit from beta-alanine supplementation, and vegetarians could possibly benefit more than non-vegetarians, although no studies have compared the two groups. Now Foods makes a vegan beta-alanine supplement.

Beta-alanine appears to be safe in amounts of 6 grams per day for up to ten weeks, although some people have reported mild numbness or tingling.

AMENORRHEA IN ATHLETES

Amenorrhea, or a loss of menstruation, may affect as many as 65 percent of young women who are long-distance runners. Hormone changes, inadequate calorie intake, and low body weight are all thought to contribute to the problem. At one time, vegetarian women were believed to be at higher risk for developing amenorrhea, but that no longer seems to be the case.

Amenorrhea correlates strongly with poor bone health. Even though weight-bearing exercise protects bones, it doesn't seem to compensate for the reduced bone formation that is seen in women who stop menstruating.

The best treatment for amenorrhea is to decrease exercise, increase calories, and, if necessary, increase body weight. Increasing calories by 200 to 300 per day and not exercising for one day per week is a reasonable approach to restoring a normal menstrual cycle. It is also crucial for all female athletes to meet recommendations for calcium and vitamin D. Vegans may need to use calcium supplements to boost intake of this essential mineral.

GUIDELINES FOR VEGAN ATHLETES: A QUICK SUMMARY

Strength Training

- Pay attention to hunger signals to make sure you are consuming adequate calories. Inadequate calorie intake can hinder muscle growth.
- Protein needs may be higher, especially in the early stages of strength training. Aim for 1.3 to 1.8 grams of protein per kilogram (0.6 to 0.8 grams of protein per pound) of body weight.
- Eating a high-protein snack after working out can increase muscle mass.
- Don't let fat intake drop too low. Eat a diet that provides 20 to 35 percent of its calories as fat. Trained athletes may perform better at the higher end of this range.
- Some weight lifters may benefit from creatine supplements.

Endurance Training

- Protein needs may be highest at the earlier stages of training. Vegan athletes should aim for 1.3 to 1.55 grams per kilogram (0.6 to 0.7 grams per pound) of body weight. The higher calorie intake of endurance athletes usually makes it easy to meet protein needs.
- Consume between 20 and 35 percent of calories from fat. The higher end of the range may be optimal for trained athletes.
- Female endurance athletes should have their iron levels checked periodically.

SAMPLE MENU

Sample Menu for a 180-Pound Male Weight Lifter

Endurance athletes are likely to meet protein needs easily because of their higher calorie intake. Those engaged in weight training may need to put a greater emphasis on protein-rich foods. The following menu demonstrates one way in which those needs can be met.

BREAKFAST
- 1 ½ cups tofu
- 3 slices whole-wheat toast
- 1 tablespoon vegan margarine
- 2 tablespoons fruit preserves
- 1 cup orange juice

SNACK
- ½ cup trail mix (half nuts, half dried fruit)

LUNCH
- 2 whole-wheat pita pockets
- 1 cup hummus
- Salad greens with vinaigrette dressing
- 1 cup fresh fruit

SNACK
- Whole-grain English muffin
- 2 tablespoons peanut butter

DINNER
- 2 cups quinoa
- 1 cup barbecued seitan
- 2 cups steamed kale with 2 teaspoons olive oil

SNACK
- 1 cup vanilla soy yogurt
- ¼ cup granola

- 3,500 calories (18–19 calories per pound)
- 126 grams of protein (1.5 grams per kilogram or 0.7 grams per pound of body weight)

CHAPTER 15

IS IT SAFE TO EAT SOY?

Tofu, soymilk, miso, and tempeh have been staples of Asian cuisine for centuries. But soybeans have also given rise to a new generation of products that include substitutes for ground beef, chicken nuggets, luncheon slices, hotdogs, cheese, and sour cream.

There is no doubt about it: Both the traditional and the more modern soyfoods have made it easier than ever to be vegan. And aside from their practical benefits, soyfoods offer some unique health advantages— but there have also been questions about their safety.

It's no small topic: Approximately 2,000 soy-related papers appear in medical and scientific journals every year. This chapter, which looks at both the potential benefits of soy as well as some of the more controversial issues, is meant to help clarify the findings so you can make an informed decision about how these foods fit into your diet.

SOY NUTRITION

Soybeans are unique among legumes. They're higher in protein and fat and lower in carbohydrate than other beans. While much of the fat is the polyunsaturated omega-6 type, soybeans are one of the few good plant sources of omega-3 fatty acids. The carbohydrate in soybeans is composed largely of oligosaccharides, which are sugars that stimulate the growth of healthy bacteria.

The soybean's claim to fame, though, is its protein content. Soy protein is highly digestible and its amino acid pattern closely matches human requirements. It is considered comparable to proteins from animal foods and, according to the protein rating system that ranks proteins based on their amino acid pattern and digestibility, is the most highly rated of all plant proteins.[1] Soybeans are also good sources of iron, potassium, folate, and sometimes calcium. Although they contain absorption inhibitors like phytate and oxalate, iron[2] and calcium[3,4] are both easily absorbed from soyfoods. In fact, the iron in soy is present in a form called ferritin, which makes these foods somewhat unique.[5] Preliminary research suggests that ferritin iron may be very well absorbed. The calcium in fortified soymilk is absorbed as easily as calcium from cow's milk.[6,7]

Soy Isoflavones

Soybeans are the only commonly consumed food that contains nutritionally relevant amounts of isoflavones. These are members of a larger group of compounds called phytoestrogens, or plant estrogens.

Isoflavones bind to the same receptors in the body—a necessary step for biological action—that bind the hormone estrogen. This has led to one of the biggest misconceptions about isoflavones—namely, that they are the same as estrogen. They're not. Instead isoflavones are among a group of complex compounds called SERMS, or selective estrogen receptor modulators.[8]

It's the word "selective" that describes how different isoflavones are from estrogen. There are two types of estrogen receptors in cells, and estrogen binds equally to both of them. But isoflavones preferentially bind to one type of estrogen receptor and, as a result, they can act very differently from estrogen in some parts of the body. Depending upon which type of receptor dominates in a given tissue, SERMs can have estrogen-like effects—or anti-estrogenic effects or no effects at all.

Isoflavones are natural SERMS, but some drugs used to treat cancer and osteoporosis are also SERMS. For example, the osteoporosis drug raloxifene has estrogen-like effects on bone and possibly on LDL-cholesterol, two areas in which estrogen is protective and beneficial. But raloxifene may have anti-estrogenic effects in the breast, thereby reducing breast cancer risk.[9]

One issue regarding isoflavones may be of particular interest to vegetarians and vegans. The way in which isoflavones are metabolized can differ significantly among individuals and this could impact their health effects. For example, one type of isoflavone is metabolized by intestinal bacteria to a compound called equol, which may be beneficial to health. But only around 25 percent of westerners have equol-producing bacteria in their intestines, compared to roughly 50 percent of Asians.[10] Interestingly, a small study found that vegetarians are more likely than meat-eaters to be equol producers.[11] Therefore, vegetarians and vegans may stand to gain more from consuming soyfoods than those eating a more typical American diet.

SOY AND HEALTH

Heart Disease

Because soyfoods are low in saturated fat, using them in place of meat and dairy can reduce blood-cholesterol levels by as much as 3 to 6 percent.[12] But there is much more to the story about soy and heart health. The protein in soy has a direct effect on blood-cholesterol levels, and simply adding it to the diet has been shown to lower cholesterol levels.[13] Moreover, studies of people in the United Kingdom[14] and Asia[15] have linked higher soy protein consumption to lower cholesterol levels.

Most studies show that it takes as much as 25 grams of soy protein per day (the amount in about three servings of traditional soyfoods) to lower cholesterol, but lower amounts could be beneficial too. The effect is modest—about a 4-percent reduction in LDL-cholesterol—but that can be enough to reduce heart disease risk by as much as 10 percent over time.[16,17]

The impact of soy is much greater when it is teamed up with other heart-healthy components. The Portfolio Diet is an experimental approach that derives much of its protein from soy and includes plenty of fiber, nuts, and foods fortified with plant sterols (compounds with natural cholesterol-lowering properties). This approach lowers LDL-cholesterol by nearly 30 percent; it's as effective for reducing cholesterol as some drug therapies.[18] Also, soy protein may impact LDL-cholesterol in ways that make it less harmful and less likely to cause clogged arteries.[19]

And there is reason to believe that soy has other coronary benefits that have nothing to do with its protein or fat content or, for that matter, blood-cholesterol levels. Several Chinese and Japanese studies show that people who consume two servings of soyfoods per day are only half as likely to have heart disease compared to those who consume marginal amounts of soy.[20–23] That's a dramatic difference—far more than could be due to the cholesterol-lowering effects of soyfoods. These additional protective effects may be related not to protein or fat but to isoflavones, which may directly improve the health of the arteries.[24] Since many people who suffer heart attacks don't have elevated cholesterol, these additional potential benefits of soyfoods could mean that they offer protection even for people with low cholesterol levels.

Soy and Bone Health

Since estrogen therapy reduces bone loss and fracture risk in post-menopausal women, there has been a great deal of interest in determining whether isoflavones have the same benefits.[25] More than twenty-five clinical trials have looked at the effects of isoflavones on bone health, mostly in postmenopausal women.[26–28] Some have found that soyfoods, soy protein, and isoflavone supplements improve bone-mineral density, but others haven't shown any benefit.

It may be that soy isoflavones simply aren't protective. Remember that isoflavones are SERMS, which means they don't always act like estrogen, so they may not have estrogen-like effects on bones. Or possibly the isoflavone supplements used in the studies are less effective than actual soyfoods because compounds sometimes act differently when they are isolated from a food. Here's one other possible explanation: It could be that a protective effect requires lifelong soy consumption. The clinical studies involved postmenopausal women who typically consumed soy for no more than two years. In contrast, epidemiologic studies of 35,000 subjects in Singapore and 24,000 subjects in China found that women with the highest soyfood consumption—approximately two servings per day—were one-third less likely to fracture a bone.[29,30] It is reasonable to presume that these women consumed soyfoods throughout their lives.

Since most soyfoods are rich in protein and many are good sources of calcium, they certainly promote bone health. But whether soy isoflavones add additional protection remains to be seen.

Hot Flashes

Although hot flashes are relatively common among western women as they go through menopause, women in Japan seldom report having them. One reason might be that they benefit from the estrogen-like effects of isoflavones. Nearly fifty studies have examined the effect of soyfoods and different types of isoflavone supplements on hot flash incidence and/or severity and, again, the results are inconsistent.[31–33] In some studies, women had considerable relief from hot flashes; in others the relief was minor or nonexistent. The varied responses might be due in part to the fact that individuals metabolize isoflavones differently.[34] Some women may have metabolic advantages that allow them to experience relief with isoflavones.

An alternative explanation is that some soy products may be more effective at minimizing the effects of hot flashes than others. In one comprehensive analysis of seventeen studies, the supplements that were most effective were those that had an isoflavone pattern similar to soybeans. For example, soyfoods are typically rich in an isoflavone called genistein; supplements in which at least half of their total isoflavone content was in the form of genistein were very effective in studies. Consuming an amount of isoflavones that is equivalent to approximately two servings of soyfoods consistently reduced the frequency and severity of hot flashes by about 50 percent. For women who have as many as seven to ten hot flashes per day, a 50 percent reduction can provide significant relief.

Breast Cancer

In 1990, the National Cancer Institute began looking at soyfoods and isoflavones as a possible way to reduce the risk of cancer.[35] While their interest was in all cancers, they placed a particular focus on breast cancer. Most breast tumors are stimulated by estrogen, and there was evidence early on that isoflavones could have anti-estrogenic effects on breast tissue.[36,37] In addition, the historically low rates of breast cancer in Asia suggested that there was something about an Asian lifestyle that was protective.[38]

Twenty years later, the effect of soy consumption on cancer risk remains a question mark. Soy detractors have suggested that soy is not protective and may, in fact, be harmful for women at risk for breast cancer. However, the most recent evidence, as we'll see below, suggests that soyfoods may actually be beneficial for breast cancer patients.

Certain types of studies in mice have raised questions about soy consumption for women who have estrogen-positive breast tumors (the kind that are stimulated by estrogen).[39] But humans and mice have very different physiologic responses to isoflavones, which means the relevance of these findings to humans is uncertain. Furthermore, even in the animal studies, whole soyfoods didn't have adverse effects.[40] More importantly, studies of women show that neither whole soyfoods nor isoflavone supplements have harmful effects on indicators of breast cancer risk, such as breast cell proliferation and breast tissue density.[41] The position of the American Cancer Society is that breast cancer patients can safely consume up to three servings of traditional soyfoods daily.[42]

In fact, new epidemiologic studies show that women who consume soyfoods after a diagnosis of breast cancer have an improved prognosis. A Chinese study involving more than 5,000 women with breast cancer found that those who consumed the most soy after their diagnosis—about two servings per day—were about one-third less likely to have a cancer recurrence or to die from their disease compared with women who consumed little soy.[43] Eating soy was found to be as protective as taking the breast cancer drug tamoxifen.

A much smaller study, also from China, showed similar findings in postmenopausal breast cancer patients.[44] This study also found that soyfood consumption enhanced the efficacy of one of the most commonly used types of breast cancer drugs. Because these were epidemiologic studies, and because they involved Chinese women who almost certainly had consumed soy throughout their lives, we have to use care in interpreting the results for western women. But the evidence increasingly suggests that soy is safe and even potentially beneficial for women with breast cancer.

This, of course, raises an important question: Could adding soy to the diet help prevent breast cancer? Unfortunately the clinical studies suggest that adults who add soy to their diet don't lower their risk. In contrast, there is impressive evidence that modest soy intake (as little as one serving of soyfoods per day) during childhood and/or the teen years reduces the risk for breast cancer later in life by as much as 50 percent.[45,46] Since girls in Asian countries grow up eating soyfoods, this may in part explain the lower breast cancer rates in these populations.

At present, we can say that in healthy women, soyfoods don't raise breast cancer risk, and, while it remains speculative, they may offer benefits for women who have had breast cancer. The most promising findings, though, are that young girls who consume soy could have a lower lifetime risk of getting breast cancer.

Prostate Cancer

There is reason to believe that soy lowers the risk for prostate cancer. First, the rates of prostate cancer are low in soyfood-consuming countries compared to western populations.[47] Asian men who consume higher amounts of soy are about 30 percent less likely to develop prostate cancer than those who consume little soy.[48] Recent clinical research involving prostate cancer patients suggests that isoflavones might inhibit the spread of prostate cancer. This suggests that soyfoods may turn out to be useful for both the treatment and prevention of prostate cancer.[49] Since prostate tumors are slow growing and are typically diagnosed late in life, anything that delays tumor onset or growth can profoundly impact prostate cancer mortality. As we mentioned in Chapter 12, there is evidence that a diet high in dairy products could raise the risk for prostate cancer. So it may be that men who adopt a vegan diet and replace milk with soymilk will have added protection against prostate cancer.

Cognitive Function

Since estrogen appears to help maintain cognitive function in older women, there is speculation that soy isoflavones could have a similar effect. However, results from a study of Japanese men living in Hawaii—the Honolulu Heart Study—showed that those who ate the most tofu exhibited more signs of mental decline in their seventies through their nineties.[50] The study wasn't designed to look specifically at cognitive function, and the researchers measured the intake of only a small number of foods—two factors that limit interpretation of the findings. Also, the way in which soy intake was assessed changed over the course of the study. This too may have influenced conclusions about how much soy the men ate. In another study, which looked at women in Indonesia, tofu consumption was linked to memory loss, but tempeh—a fermented soy product that is a staple of Indonesian diets—had the opposite effect. The reason for the difference could be that in Indonesia, tofu has been typically preserved with formaldehyde, a toxic compound that can harm brain function. Recently, there have been successful efforts to prevent the use of formaldehyde in tofu production in Indonesia.[51]

Another study in Hong Kong found no effect—positive or negative—of soyfood consumption on cognitive function.[52] More importantly, most clinical studies have shown improvements in some aspects of cognitive function with soy consumption.[53]

Thyroid Function

Many foods, including soyfoods, millet, cruciferous vegetables, and some herbs, contain goitrogens. These compounds interfere with thyroid function (and in extreme cases can cause an enlarged thyroid, which is called a goiter). Generally, they cause problems only in parts of the world where iodine intake is low, since iodine is an essential nutrient needed for thyroid function. The effects of iodine deficiency can be made worse if the diet is high in goitrogens. For western vegans, this shouldn't be a problem as long as your diet includes sufficient iodine—an easy task if you use small amounts of iodized table salt every day or take an iodine supplement.

Concerns about the effects of isoflavones on thyroid function derive mostly from studies in animals.[54] In humans, the evidence clearly shows that neither soyfoods nor isoflavones adversely affect thyroid function in healthy people.[55] This research includes two recently published longer-term studies, which took place over three years and found no adverse effects of high doses of isoflavones on thyroid function. One of these studies assessed extremely sensitive indicators of thyroid function, much more sensitive than simply measuring thyroid hormones, and still it found no adverse effects.[56] In most studies, isoflavone intake was quite a bit higher than what Japanese people typically consume, and there was no ill effect on thyroid function.

High-fiber foods, including soyfoods, can reduce absorption of the synthetic thyroid hormones used by people with hypothyroidism. This is why synthetic thyroid drugs should be consumed on an empty stomach. The key to balancing intake with medication is to be consistent in consumption—that is, eat roughly the same amount of soyfoods every day—which is also important for the goitrogenic vegetables.

Finally, approximately 10 percent of older people have subclinical hypothyroidism—a condition that lies somewhere between having a healthy thyroid and hypothyroidism. As a precaution, people with this condition should have their thyroid function monitored if they decide to change their intake of soyfoods because this is an area that hasn't been well-researched.

Reproductive Health and Feminization

Stories that make their way around the Internet about the negative impact on testosterone and feminizing effects of isoflavones are not supported by the research. A comprehensive analysis published in 2010 showed that neither soyfoods nor isoflavones affect testosterone levels.[57] Similarly, there is no evidence that soyfoods or isoflavones, when consumed in amounts even greatly exceeding typical Japanese intake, have any effect on estrogen levels in men.[58]

In a study of soy intake and sperm characteristics, researchers found that sperm counts in men with higher soy intakes did not differ from those who ate no soy. Men who ate more soy had lower sperm concentrations, but this was partly due to a higher semen volume.[59]

In contrast, clinical studies show no effects of isoflavones on sperm or semen, even when isoflavone intakes are ten times greater than what Japanese men typically consume.[60] In fact, as a result of their findings, one research team suggested that isoflavones may be a treatment for low sperm concentration.[61]

Soyfoods have been a part of Asian diets for centuries and there has never been any indication that they affect reproduction in these populations. Current research on this issue supports what history has long shown.

HOW MUCH AND
WHAT KIND OF SOY TO EAT

It's always smart to build a diet on a foundation of whole, unprocessed foods and to include a variety of foods in every meal. Where do soy-foods fit in? We can look to traditional Asian diets for guidance, stay-ing mindful that a couple of common beliefs about Asian soyfood consumption—that soy is consumed mostly as fermented foods and used only as a condiment—are both wrong.

Fermented foods, such as miso, were the first soyfoods consumed in Asian countries, but that in no way means that people in Asia con-sume mostly fermented soyfoods. Nonfermented foods like tofu have been a part of Asian diets for at least 1,000 years and continue to play a significant role in these cultures. In China, soymilk and tofu make up the bulk of the soyfoods in diets. In Japan, about half the soy intake is from the fermented foods miso and natto and the other half comes from unfermented foods like tofu.[62]

A number of vegan foods, including veggie burgers and other meat analogs, are made from isolated soy protein or soy protein concen-trate. They have been the target of some criticism because they are highly processed, but there is actually nothing unsafe about them. In fact, most of the studies on the protein quality of soy—which looked at the ability of soy to support protein balance in humans—used iso-lated soy proteins.[63]

Surveys show that people in Japan and urban areas of China such as Shanghai typically consume around 1½ servings of soyfoods per day, although there is a wide range of intakes.[64] It's interesting to note that some of the health benefits associated with soy have been seen in people who consume the most soyfoods.

There is no requirement to include soy in your diet, but there is no reason to avoid these foods either. Since variety is an important factor in planning healthy diets, we recommend limiting soyfoods to three to four servings per day. Veggie burgers and other foods made from soy protein can be part of an overall healthy diet, but to get the full nutritional—and culinary—benefits of soy, be sure to explore some of the more traditional foods such as tofu and tempeh. The Soyfoods Primer on pages 119–123 can help familiarize you with these foods.

ISOFLAVONE, PROTEIN, AND CALORIE CONTENT OF SOYFOODS

Soyfood	Isoflavones (in milligrams)	Protein (in grams)	Calories
Tofu			
Tofu, firm, ½ cup	31.5	10	88
Tofu, regular, ½ cup	29.3	10	94
Silken tofu, ½ cup	34.6	8.6	77
Natto, ½ cup	52	15.6	186
Soymilk, 1 cup	11.6	4.56	65
Miso, 1 tablespoon	6.4	1.75	30
Tempeh, ½ cup	36.1	15.3	160
Soynuts, ¼ cup	55	17	194
Soybeans, ½ cup cooked	47	14.3	149
Soybeans, green, ½ cup cooked	17.7	15.7	180
Isolated soy protein, 1 ounce	28.7	22.6	95
Soy protein concentrate, 1 ounce	3.5–28.6 (varies depending on processing)	16.2	93
Soyflour, full fat, ¼ cup	37.4	7.2	92
Soyflour, defatted, ¼ cup	32.8	11.7	82.5

CHAPTER 16

WHY VEGAN?

Modern farming methods force animals to live in conditions most people cannot imagine. The abuses that we describe in this chapter are not unusual in the world of today's agricultural industry. Many are standard and routine and are depicted in the trade magazines of animal agriculture. We've also included observations from some of the undercover investigations that have given Americans a look at the shocking conditions—some legal, some not—under which animal foods are produced.

We think you'll agree that the facts make a compelling case for going vegan.

Some of the information in this book comes straight from publications of the agriculture industry, but much of it is the result of undercover investigations by four national nonprofit organizations. More information, including videos of many of these investigations, can be found on their websites:

▸ The Humane Society of the United States (HSUS)
　www.humanesociety.org
▸ People for the Ethical Treatment of Animals (PETA)
　www.peta.org
▸ Mercy For Animals (MFA)
　www.mercyforanimals.org
▸ Compassion Over Killing (COK)
　www.cok.net

You can also view videos of factory farming investigations on the Vegan Outreach website: www.veganoutreach/video.org

---

LIFE ON A MODERN FARM

Films and photos produced by the agricultural industry show pictures of clean facilities and animals who appear well cared for and in good health. Investigations by animal protection advocates reveal a different story: filthy conditions, birds missing feathers, and animals with sores and injuries. While it's hard to say what the average farm is like, animal protection advocates document squalid farms on a regular basis. They also frequently find cases of wanton cruelty against farm animals despite the industry's insistence that such incidents are rare and highly unusual.

People don't like to think that farm or slaughterhouse employees would intentionally cause an animal to suffer. The truth is that those whose job it is to "process" thousands of animals an hour are likely to develop an insensitivity toward the "product." In a 2008 undercover investigation of Aviagen Turkeys Inc., one of the world's leading turkey breeding companies, PETA documented employees stomping on turkeys' heads, punching turkeys, hitting them on the head with a can of spray paint and pliers, and striking the turkeys' heads against metal scaffolding. Workers also shoved feces and feed into turkeys' mouths and held turkeys' heads under water.[1]

When a supervisor was questioned about the treatment, he responded: "Every once in a while, everybody gets agitated and has to kill a bird."

While the industry might downplay the significance of certain practices, they don't deny the use of many of the systems that we talk about in this chapter. Almost all of the methods used on different factory farms have three common elements—and all are aimed at maintaining high efficiency and low costs:

1. *Factory farms maximize the number of animals who can be raised in a given amount of space.* Confined animals save on space, and they also can't move much, which reduces their feed requirements.

(Manipulating lighting reduces feed requirements as well.) Egg-laying hens are housed in cages so small they can't stretch their wings. Breeding pigs typically can't turn around in their small crates.

The factory farming industry doesn't deny the existence of cramped conditions. They are regularly depicted in industry journals and magazines where industry representatives insist that these conditions are not cruel and that they are necessary. Farmers insist that the system wouldn't be viable if it didn't protect the health and well-being of animals. But the truth is that letting some animals die due to overcrowding is more economical than allocating more space to keep them healthy.

2. *Factory farms increase growth and production through genetics, hormones, and pesticides.* Animals grow (or produce eggs and milk) at unnatural rates. This takes a toll on their bodies and many farm animals become injured, inflamed, or arthritic. After a few years of nonstop calf and milk production, dairy cows' bodies are so abused that often they can barely walk. They sometimes have to be kicked and prodded to the killing floor.

3. *Factory farms weed out slow-producing animals.* Weak or sick animals may simply die in their cage or crate. But those who are not producing well may be sent to slaughter or are sometimes killed on the farm. Undercover investigations have shown some of these weakened animals being beaten to death.

EGG-LAYING HENS

The life of an egg-laying hen begins at the hatchery. Within minutes of emerging from their shells, male chicks are separated out and killed. In 2009, Mercy For Animals (MFA) went undercover at the world's largest hatchery for egg-laying hens, Hy-Line International, in Spencer, Iowa. They found thousands of male chicks being thrown into grinding machines, which is a routine means of chick disposal. The tiny birds are tossed by a spinning auger before being torn apart by the high-pressure macerator. In other hatcheries, live male chicks are simply loaded into dumpsters and left to suffocate or die.

The female chicks have one-third to one-half of their beaks cut off. This keeps the chickens from pecking each other in the extremely cramped cages in which they will spend their entire adult lives. Their beaks are highly sensitive to pain and some studies show that the pain lasts for as long as five to six weeks.[2]

When they arrive at the warehouse, four to six (and sometimes more) chicks are placed in a cage that is the size of a typical microwave oven. They live on wire, which cuts into their feet and scrapes their feathers, and as they grow into full-sized chickens, the birds become so cramped that they can't extend their wings.

With thousands of chickens living on a typical farm, no attention is paid to individual birds. Many die from dehydration or starvation if they become caught in the wires, if their toenails grow around the wires, or if the mechanized food or water delivery system malfunctions. Others die from inhalation of ammonia from the manure pits below the cages. Hens are bred to produce such large eggs that sometimes these eggs pull the tube they are supposed to move through right out of the hen's body. This is called a prolapsed oviduct, and it results in hemorrhage, infection, and death.

Hens live in these conditions for one to two years or until their egg production begins to decline and they are removed from their cages and killed. If the hens have become stuck to the cages, they are ripped out, and because their bones are often brittle from high egg production and inadequate calcium, many of them suffer fractures in the process.[3]

Laying hens may be sent to slaughter, but they are often in such poor condition that they can't be used by the food industry. On one farm, "spent" hens (as they are called by the industry) were tossed into a wood chipper for disposal.

Carbon dioxide gassing is the more common means of killing spent hens. Gas concentration of 30 percent or more is necessary to kill the birds, and research has shown that at this level, birds will feel pain and distress, probably associated with suffocation.

Once the hens have been removed from the warehouses, the manure is plowed out of the buildings and new chicks are brought in to start the cycle again.

UNDERCOVER INVESTIGATIONS OF EGG FARMS

Michael Foods is one of the nation's largest egg producers, supplying eggs to several national restaurant chains including Dunkin' Donuts. In 2009, an investigator from Compassion Over Killing (COK) worked inside one of Michael Foods' factory farms and documented numerous abuses:

- hens immobilized in the wires of their cages, unable to reach food or water
- decomposing and "mummified" corpses left in cages with live birds (who were producing eggs for human consumption)
- an employee decapitating a hen
- birds suffering from overcrowding, severe feather loss, and untreated injuries

Upon viewing the film, Dr. Ian Duncan, chair of animal welfare in the Department of Animal and Poultry Science at the University of Guelph in Canada, said that the conditions of the carcasses suggested that some birds had been dead in their cages for well over a week. The hens may have been unable to reach food and water and died slowly from dehydration and starvation.[4]

Over the following two years, MFA found similar conditions at two other large egg farms: Quality Egg of New England in Turner, Maine,[5] and Norco Ranch in Menifee, California.[6] Some of what they observed was typical for egg farms—birds confined in wire cages so tiny they couldn't walk, stretch their wings, or engage in basic behaviors. But they also saw birds with bloody, open wounds and hens being kicked by workers into manure pits or being thrown into trash cans while still alive. In both places, workers were observed killing birds by swinging them in an arc to break their necks.

BIRDS RAISED FOR MEAT

Like hens who lay eggs for human consumption, "breeders" or meat chickens, and sometimes turkeys, have part of their beaks removed when they are very young.[7] Farmers may also trim the bills of ducks (sometimes using scissors).[8] The toes of turkeys are often cut off without painkillers to prevent scratching.[9] In PETA's investigation of Aviagen Turkeys, they found hens whose beaks were cut with pliers and birds who had collapsed and died of exhaustion or heart attacks.[10]

Birds may become lame and unable to walk because they have been genetically selected to grow abnormally large. A 2003 COK investigation of a chicken farm found chickens who could not walk due to leg deformities, as well as chickens trapped in the feeders. In studies on the effects of these deformities, lame birds are more likely than non-lame birds to eat feed that is laced with painkillers, an indication that they are in pain. The COK investigation also revealed that the levels of ammonia in the air were high enough to cause eye and trachea lesions in birds.[11]

PÂTÉ DE FOIE GRAS

Pâté de foie gras, made from the fattened liver of ducks or geese, is not a significant part of most American diets, but it is one example of the extreme cruelty that is legal in factory farming. To quickly produce fattened livers, ducks and geese are force-fed through tubes placed in their throats.

In 2008, an investigator from COK videotaped conditions inside Hudson Valley Foie Gras in Ferndale, New York. The video shows foot-long tubes being shoved down the throats of ducks to force food into their stomachs.[12]

PIGS

The majority of breeder pigs spend years in pens so narrow that they can't turn around.[13] They usually live on metal grates or concrete floors amidst urine and feces. Crated pigs develop repetitive behaviors like banging their heads against the cages and biting the metal rails. About 20 percent are killed each year due to lameness.[14]

The non-breeding pigs raised for meat live in somewhat less cramped quarters and can turn around. But conditions are still restricted and dark, and the air is filled with the scent of ammonia. Because of ammonia levels, respiratory problems are the leading killer of pigs grown for meat.[15] Like birds, they are bred to grow faster than their bodies can handle, and many become lame and eventually are unable to walk.

PETA and MFA undertook three undercover investigations of pig farms between 2007 and 2009, and they found numerous abuses. Workers dragged injured pigs out of the facility by their snouts, ears, and legs before killing them with a captive bolt gun, and employees cut off piglets' tails and castrated them without using painkillers.

On one farm, a supervisor admitted on video that he violently beat pigs. Other acts of wanton cruelty included workers beating pigs, jabbing them in their eyes, shoving a cane up one of the sow's vaginas, and spraying paint into the nose of a nursing sow. Young pigs who had been gassed improperly were still alive when the gas container was opened. Piglets were tossed through the air among workers. Pigs with cysts, sores, and uterine prolapses received no medical treatment.[16–18]

DAIRY COWS

A majority of dairy cows are kept in large feedlots, where they live on a layer of mud and feces and among swarms of flies. To keep milk production high, cows are impregnated repeatedly. Their calves are taken from them soon after birth, often causing extreme anguish to the mother cow and her newborn.

According to USDA statistics, the average dairy cow's milk production has increased from two to ten tons per year since 1940.[19] Their bodies are so stressed by this hyper-production that by the time they are sent to slaughter (once production has declined), many "go down" and are unable to walk into the slaughterhouse. They are then dragged to a "dead pile" and left to die.

In September 2009, PETA released undercover footage of a Pennsylvania dairy facility that supplies the Land O'Lakes company. Over the course of several months, the investigation documented filthy conditions for cows on the farm, such as pens that were filled inches deep with excrement, which caused foot and hoof problems. Some cows were so ill that they had collapsed. The video footage shows cows struggling to walk or unable to stand up. Calves rescued from the farm had pneumonia, "manure scald," ringworm, pinkeye, and parasites. Some cows suffered respiratory distress and had pus-filled nasal discharge streaming down their faces.[20] In order to make milking easier, the cows' tails were amputated by tightly binding them with elastic bands, causing the skin and tissue to slowly die and slough off, and leaving the animals unable to swat away flies. In one case, workers were told to wrap an elastic band around a cow's gangrenous, infected teat in order to amputate it. The cow's condition deteriorated for eleven days before she finally died.

In 2009, at Willet Dairy in Locke, New York, the largest dairy farm in the state, an MFA undercover video shows cows with udders that are shockingly large due to the production of an unnatural volume of milk, and cows with open wounds, prolapsed uteruses, pus-filled infections, and swollen joints. Some were too weak to stand, and dead cows and calves were found on the premises.[21]

VEAL CALVES

Male calves born on dairy farms are typically taken from their mothers right after birth. Most are raised for "milk-fed" veal.[22] They are tethered in stalls where they can't turn around. This lack of movement and their iron-deficient liquid diet makes the meat from these animals more tender and pale. The calves live this way for sixteen to eighteen weeks before being sent to slaughter.

About 15 percent of calves are slaughtered when they are just a few days or weeks old for "bob veal."[23] Often, these newborns are too weak to walk. A 2009 HSUS investigation of a Vermont "bob veal" slaughterhouse showed workers kicking and electrically prodding newborn calves who struggled to walk to slaughter. They threw water in some of the calves' faces to make the electrical prodding more painful. The workers were also filmed cutting portions of skin off still-living calves in front of the USDA inspector.[24] Improper stunning of the calves meant that some were conscious when they were shackled by one leg and hung upside down to have their throats slit.

BEEF CATTLE

The beef industry paints an idyllic picture of steers grazing contentedly on grassy hillsides. These cattle may be able to move freely, but their lives are not without pain and trauma. Cattle are hot-iron branded and castrated with no anesthetic. And after several months of life on the ranch, the animals are trucked to large feedlots, where they live in pens and are fattened on grains. Harris Ranch in Coalinga, California, holds more than 100,000 beef cows for fattening. They live on a layer of dirt mixed with feces, and the stench can be smelled from miles away.

Ranching impacts the lives of many wild animals as well, especially those that prey on cattle. In 2008, 89,300 coyotes were killed by the USDA Animal Plant and Health Inspection Services' Wildlife Services Department to protect cattle. Other animals, particularly bison from Yellowstone National Park, that threaten to pass disease to cattle are often killed by government employees or hunters.

TRANSPORT

As slaughterhouses have consolidated, animals are trucked long distances to slaughter. They are typically not fed for many hours at a time

and are subject to extreme heat and cold, as well as highway accidents. At least one trucker admitted that he leaves cattle on a truck
for up to sixty hours without water. Many animals die in transport or
are too weak to walk when they arrive at the slaughterhouse.[25]

Animals that cannot walk are treated horribly. They may be repeatedly shocked with electricity or dragged by chains. Some are pushed by
a backhoe and dumped in a dead pile, where they die a slow death.

SLAUGHTER

With the exception of kosher and halal slaughter, mammals are by law
to be rendered unconscious before they are killed. This is often done
with a shot from a captive bolt pistol. Studies show that the shooter
misses the mark in a small but consistent percentage of cases. The
American Meat Institute considers a 95-percent stun rate acceptable.[26]
According to a 2008 survey, 25 percent of beef slaughter plants obtained a level of stunning of 95 percent to 99 percent on the first at-
tempt. But while the percentage of animals who are not rendered
unconscious on the first try is small, the actual number isn't. It may be
true that "only" 1 to 5 percent of all cattle are insufficiently stunned,
but that means that as many as 345,000 to 1.7 million cows per year
must be stunned more than once—or they remain conscious during at
least part of the slaughter process.[27]

Slaughterhouse consultant Temple Grandin said, "Unfortunately,
effective stunning and reducing skull fracturing [to prevent the spread
of mad cow disease via brain tissue entering the flesh] are two opposite
goals. As the amount of damage to the skull is reduced, placement of
the shot must become more and more precise to achieve instantaneous insensibility. Shooting on a slight angle may result in failure to
induce instantaneous insensibility."[28]

In "Modern Meat: A Brutal Harvest," a 2001 article from the
Washington Post, the reality of insufficient stunning was made graphi-
cally clear:

It takes twenty-five minutes to turn a live steer into steak at the modern slaughterhouse where Ramon Moreno works. For twenty years, his post was "second-legger," a job that entails cutting hocks off carcasses as they whirl past at a rate of 309 an hour. The cattle were supposed to be dead before they got to Moreno. But too often they weren't.

"They blink. They make noises," he said softly. "The head moves, the eyes are wide and looking around."

Still Moreno would cut. On bad days, he says, dozens of animals reached his station clearly alive and conscious. Some would survive as far as the tail cutter, the belly ripper, the hide puller.

"They die," said Moreno, "piece by piece."[29]

Fast line speeds at the slaughterhouse are typically to blame for the fact that animals are often conscious as they move down the line. Workers are under too much pressure to keep the line moving and cannot take the time to worry about a still-conscious animal who has slipped by.

In testimony before the U.S. House of Representatives Oversight and Government Reform Committee, Dr. Dean Wyatt, a USDA public health supervisory veterinarian, said that he saw calves being dragged and thrown and left to die without food or water and animals being killed without stunning. Dr. Wyatt testified that he had been directed by his superiors at the agency to "drastically cut back" the time spent ensuring that animals destined for food were treated humanely. He was threatened with termination, and other inspectors were chastised, reprimanded, and demoted for reporting violations.[30]

Poultry Slaughter

Birds (and rabbits) are not required to be stunned or unconscious when they are slaughtered. Although birds' heads are usually run through water that has an electric current to paralyze them for easier handling, it's unlikely that this renders them unconscious. When their throats are cut, if the blade misses—a frequent occurrence when the process is mechanized—birds may be awake and alert when they are dropped into the scalding tank to be boiled alive. The USDA refers to birds who are still alive when they reach the scalding tank as "cadavers" and condemns them from the food supply because they contain too much blood and are discolored. USDA statistics show that over 1 million chickens and over 30,000 turkeys were condemned as cadavers in 2008.[31]

From December 2004 through February 2005, a PETA undercover investigator worked on the slaughter line of a Tyson Foods chicken processing plant in Heflin, Alabama. Using a hidden camera, he documented the treatment of the more than 100,000 chickens killed every day in the plant:

- Birds were frequently mutilated by throat-cutting machines that didn't work properly; one bird had her skin entirely torn off her chest.
- Workers were instructed to rip the heads off birds who had missed the throat-cutting machines.
- Plant employees jokingly tossed around dying birds.
- Plant managers told the investigator that it was acceptable for forty animals per shift to be scalded alive in the feather-removal tank, and no one was reprimanded when far more than forty birds suffered this fate during any given shift.[32]

Shockingly, just two years later, a PETA investigation into Tyson slaughter plants in Georgia and Tennessee showed that the abuses at this company had worsened. The investigator documented birds hung from shackles by their necks rather than their feet, birds trapped under the door at the end of the conveyor belt, and workers urinating on the conveyer belt. Supervisors were sometimes directly involved in the abuses or failed to stop them. One stated on videotape that it was acceptable to rip the heads off live birds who had been improperly shackled by the head.[33]

At the House of Raeford Farms, one of the country's largest poultry slaughterhouses, a 2007 MFA investigation found workers ripping heads off of live turkeys, birds being crushed to death beneath the wheels of trucks, and a worker punching shackled turkeys.[34]

Pig Slaughter

Prior to slaughter, pigs are typically stunned with electricity, producing a grand mal seizure. Proper stunning can take more than one try, which is very painful. In an article titled "Electric Stunning of Pigs and Sheep," Temple Grandin writes:

> To produce instantaneous, painless unconsciousness, sufficient amperage (current) must pass through the animal's brain to induce an epileptic seizure. Insufficient amperage or a current path that fails to go through the brain will be painful for the animal. It will feel a large electric shock or heart attack symptoms, even though it may be paralyzed and unable to move.[35]

Kosher and Halal Slaughter

According to the rules that govern kosher and halal slaughter, animals must be conscious when their throat is cut. In kosher slaughter, the cow should have her throat cut only once, after which she should bleed to death. But at the world's largest kosher slaughterhouse in Postville, Iowa, a 2008 PETA investigation showed workers making multiple cuts. Only months before the investigation's findings were released, the slaughterhouse had passed inspection. Temple Grandin, commenting on the investigation, noted, "The undercover video clearly showed that when they think nobody is looking, they do bad things in this plant."[36] There is a debate over whether properly performed kosher and halal slaughter actually renders the animal pain-free within the two seconds as claimed. An article on NewScientist.com reported that calves (who bleed more slowly than adults) may feel pain for up to two minutes.[37] We would encourage anyone who eats kosher meat to watch the PETA video, which includes footage of the correct way to perform kosher slaughter. The cows do appear to suffer as they bleed to death even when slaughter is performed pursuant to kosher law.[38]

FISH AND OTHER SEA CREATURES

According to experts, fish have structures that resemble the pain receptors in humans and other animals, but whether they are actually conscious of pain is subject to debate. Studies show that fish react to pain by changing their behavior, which suggests a consciousness of discomfort. It seems fair to give fish the benefit of the doubt, especially since the ways in which they are farmed, caught, and killed are particularly inhumane. All of these animals—including lobsters, crabs, and shrimp—fight for their lives to the extent that they are able.

Bottom-trawling nets pull hundreds of tons of animals from the ocean, squeezing some of them so tightly against the sides of the nets that their eyes bulge and burst out of their skulls. For hours, trapped fish are dragged along the ocean floor. When hauled out of the water, the surviving fish undergo decompression. The extreme pressure change ruptures their swim bladders, pops out their eyes, and pushes their esophagi and stomachs out through their mouths.

Commercial fishing uses drift nets that also kill tens of thousands of sea mammals such as dolphins, whales, otters, seals, and sea lions per year, as well as depleting the food sources of many of these animals.

SLOW CHANGE

There are very few laws protecting farmed animals, and some animals, such as birds, are exempt from laws regarding farmed animal slaughter. Animal agriculture interests are, on principle, opposed to regulation of agriculture and they fight vigorously to stop even the most meager improvements for animals. And they have a great deal of political clout;

most legislation to improve farmed-animal welfare must pass through agricultural committees made up of legislators from farming areas or who receive contributions from the industry.

The good news is that there have been small changes in factory farming practices over the past few years, nearly all in response to the efforts of animal protection activists. For example, since 1994, it is no longer legal to brand steers on their faces. Voters in some states have passed measures to do away with some of the cruelest confinement systems. Withholding food from chickens for two weeks to increase egg production is no longer recommended by the United Egg Producers, and the majority of farmers no longer follow this practice (although many still do). In 2009, tail docking of cows (removing part of their tail without anesthesia) was made illegal in California. In her 2008 audit, Temple Grandin reported that ten pig slaughterhouses passed with all pigs being stunned properly.

But given the extensive and routine cruelty associated with factory farming and the strength of an industry that resists even the smallest improvements, meaningful change for all farm animals is a long way off. Animal cruelty is an inherent part of factory farming. Longtime activist and Vegan.com blogger Erik Marcus put it this way:

> Many of the so-called "breakdowns" that are captured in these videos are not a result of worker incompetence or deliberate cruelty but rather stem from the design of housing systems and handling procedures. These cruelties are baked-in to the system on an industry-wide basis, and that's why every video investigation I've ever witnessed has uniformly generated the same sorts of appalling images.
>
> For instance, given the numbers of hens raised in a typical battery facility, the design of the cages, and the scarcity of employees, it's inevitable that any video shot will reveal numerous examples of animals caught in their cages or suffering from untreated medical conditions.
>
> And here's the key point: Any company that tried to unilaterally restructure by seriously boosting welfare standards, while working

within the conventional factory farming system, would face insur-mountable cost disadvantages. They'd be unable to compete and would be driven from business.

So while it's convenient to blame management or supervision, and while there are certainly brutal and callous workers at some factory farms, that's not the root of the problem. Factory farms are universally cruel by design, and these cruelties can't be removed in any way other than for the entire industry to fundamentally restructure.

If industry wants to put an end to future cruelty videos, they've got to switch to systems with more space per animal, they've got to put an end to crowded transport and hurried slaughter, and they need to hire more workers to tend fewer animals. In short, the economics that keep animal products cheap are the same economics that guarantee a constant stream of videos shining a spotlight on the industry.

This is absolutely not a matter of bad supervision: The only way agribusiness can put an end to its worst cruelties is to spend vastly more money on each animal it raises, while putting a system in place where no company can cut corners. Until then, the videos will keep right on coming.[39]

ALTERNATIVES TO FACTORY FARMS

There are many other problems associated with factory farming, related to global warming and food safety, that are beyond the scope of this book. What is clear—based on animal cruelty, environmental effects, and human health—is that factory farming must end. This then raises questions about whether there are humane options for people who wish to continue eating animal products.

There are a number of labels used on animal products that suggest the animals lived in better conditions than factory farms: "humane," "all-natural," "free range," and "organic" are some of them. You might be surprised, however, to learn that products carrying these labels almost universally come from factory-farmed animals—and from the same slaughterhouses we discussed above. For example, the slaughterhouse investigated for cruel treatment of veal calves was the same company used by organic Vermont dairy farms (see page 225).

In 2010, the Cornucopia Institute, an organic farm watchdog group, released *Scrambled Eggs: Separating Factory Farm Egg Production from Authentic Organic Agriculture*. The report was based on visits to more than 15 percent of USDA-certified organic egg farms and surveys of all name-brand and private-label industry egg companies. While organic standards include a requirement for outdoor access for animals, including laying hens, they found that "most industrial-scale producers are currently confining tens of thousands of hens inside henhouses, commonly only offering tiny concrete or wooden porches as 'outdoor access'—and getting away with it. In some cases they've used statements from veterinarians concerning hypothetical disease transmission as an excuse to offer *no outdoor access whatsoever*." (Emphasis added.)

Mark A. Kastel, the Cornucopia Institute's co-director and senior farm policy analyst, said, "[I]t's obvious that a high percentage of the eggs on the market should be labeled 'produced with organic feed' rather than bearing the USDA-certified organic logo."

For most products touted as "humanely produced," cruelty lurks behind the cheerful label. Even if free-range dairy farms provide better treatment for cows, their male calves are still taken from their mothers within hours of birth and sold for veal production. Chickens in cage-free facilities can spread their wings, but they still spend their entire lives packed by the tens of thousands into windowless warehouses. The male chicks are still killed at birth and the females are debeaked. They go to the same slaughterhouses as caged chickens.

You can read more about the various labels and what they actually mean in Farm Sanctuary's *Truth Behind the Labels* report. There is only one way to know the conditions of the animals from whom eggs, milk, and meat are derived, and that is to visit the farm where they live and the slaughterhouse where they die.

THE BETTER SOLUTION: GO VEGAN

If some of the worst factory farming abuses are eliminated through legislation, we can expect the cost of animal foods to go up and consumption to go down. Influencing the supply of animal foods in this way is an important part of dismantling animal agriculture—which is important whether you support the rights of animals or simply want to see an end to the barbarity of factory farming.

But by far the most effective and powerful way to end factory farming is to eliminate demand. And the only way to do that is to adopt a vegan lifestyle. While it's sad to think about the plight of animals on factory farms, it's empowering to know that we can choose not to contribute to their torture—and that this choice can prevent animal suffering and threaten the very existence of animal agriculture.

DO ANIMALS HAVE RIGHTS?

People who choose a vegan lifestyle because of ethical concerns for animals may have fundamental differences in their beliefs. Some believe that any use of animals is likely to involve suffering, and therefore the only humane and ethical option is to avoid all animal products. Others embrace the animal rights perspective articulated in the early 1980s by People for the Ethical Treatment of Animals: "Animals are not ours to eat, wear, or experiment on." In other words, whether or not animals are treated humanely, we don't have the right to use them for our own purposes.

Both perspectives can play critical roles in achieving the goal of eliminating animal suffering. But we believe that there is compelling reason to support the second viewpoint and that human rights can be logically extended to make the case for animal rights.

A human rights ethic suggests that no human—not just intelligent humans, but also babies, infants, and those who are mentally challenged—should be abused and used by others for whatever purpose

Catastrophes

Because huge numbers of farmed animals are confined in massive sheds on today's farms, when catastrophes strike, there is no escape. If there is a fire, flood, or tornado, these animals are doomed to burn, drown, or suffer severe injuries. Over a recent two-year period, hundreds of thousands of farm animals were the victims of these types of tragedies. In 2010, for instance, 60,000 chickens died from heat exhaustion on a North Carolina farm when the fans stopped working following a power outage. A year earlier, nearly 4,000 pigs met the same fate when a vandal turned off the fans on an Iowa farm. And on a farm in Texas, 800,000 hens died in a fire. There are many more examples of fire, flood, and transport truck accidents that cause terrifying and agonizing deaths for hundreds and thousands of animals.

they like. This raises the question about whether rights should be extended to animals. The idea that if we grant rights to humans of lesser intelligence or ability, we should also grant rights to animals is sometimes referred to as the *argument from marginal cases*. If intelligence and capability are not criteria for the possession of rights, why would animals—who have the capacity to feel fear and pain—be excluded from moral consideration? Some philosophers may reject the argument from marginal cases, but we have never known any of them to provide a compelling reason for doing so.

EXTENDING JUSTICE TO ANIMALS

In his book A *Theory of Justice*, John Rawls put forth a moral philosophy based on a hypothetical "original position." In this scenario, the person who makes the moral rules for a society does so without prior knowledge of who they will be in that society. So place yourself in this original position: You are making decisions about whose interests will be deemed important—without knowing what color your skin will be, whether you'll be a mentally-challenged person, male or female, or a cow or a chicken or a tree or a rock.

The only safe way to protect your interests is to give equal consideration to the interests of all. In this situation, you would clearly feel a strong imperative toward making things as fair as possible for everyone. Right away, we can dismiss the needs of rocks, since rocks have no needs. Plants are similar to rocks; they don't have brains or the capacity to feel pain. They can't avoid mutilation, so it would serve no purpose for them to fear it or suffer from it. (Does anyone really believe that mowing a lawn causes plants a similar agony to that of cutting off the limbs of animals or humans?)

While we don't understand everything about the needs of animals, we know that they can experience pain and fear. Is that reason enough to consider their interests? If you put yourself in the original position, knowing that you may end up as a cow or a pig, it's very likely that you would consider the interests of these animals to be important.

WHAT ABOUT INDIGENOUS PEOPLE WHO MUST KILL ANIMALS TO SURVIVE?

If someone has to kill to stay alive, can you blame them for doing so? Perhaps not, but staying alive should be the only legitimate excuse for taking the lives of others. Tradition is not a good argument, as anyone who opposes human sacrifice should agree. And doing what is *natural* is also not a good argument given how hard it is to define or know what is natural, and how few people actually seek to live in a state of nature.

These philosophies raise legitimate and powerful questions about whether we can claim any right to use animals when we don't need to and, as our book shows, a vegan diet offers such an easy, healthy and enjoyable alternative.

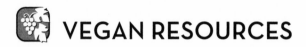 # VEGAN RESOURCES

AUTHORS' BLOGS

www.JackNorrisRD.com
www.TheVeganRD.com

RECOMMENDED SOURCES OF NUTRITION INFORMATION

www.veganhealth.org: This is Jack's comprehensive overview of vegan nutrition studies.

www.vrg.org: The Vegetarian Resource Group provides extensive information about vegan nutrition for families.

Latest in Clinical Nutrition DVDs, compiled by Michael Greger, MD: Each DVD addresses highlights of nutrition research for the year.

The Dietitian's Guide to Vegetarian Diets, 3rd ed., by Reed Mangels, Virginia Messina, and Mark Messina (Sudbury, MA: Jones and Bartlett, 2010).

Simply Vegan: Quick Vegetarian Meals, 4th ed., by Debra Wasserman and Reed Mangels (Baltimore, MD: The Vegetarian Resource Group, 2006).

VEGAN STARTER GUIDES

You can download or order free booklets on vegan nutrition and cooking from these websites:

www.veganoutreach.org/guide/
www.tryveg.com/request/
www.mercyforanimals.org/vegan-starter-kit.aspx
www.humanesociety.org/assets/pdfs/farm/gve.pdf

ONLINE VEGAN STORES

www.cosmosveganshoppe.com/
www.healthy-eating.com
www.veganessentials.com
www.veganstore.com
www.thevegetariansite.com

VEGAN NEWS AND VIEWS

www.vegan.com
www.diggingthroughthedirt.blogspot.com
www.whyveganoutreach.blogspot.com/
www.vegnews.com

VEGAN EDUCATION, ACTIVISM, AND LIFESTYLE

The Animal Activist's Handbook by Matt Ball and Bruce Friedrich (New York: Lantern Books, 2009).

Strategic Action for Animals: A Handbook on Strategic Movement Building, Organizing, and Activism for Animal Liberation by Melanie Joy (New York: Lantern Books, 2008).

Striking at the Roots: A Practical Guide to Animal Activism by Mark Hawthorne (Winchester, UK: O Books, 2007).

Thanking the Monkey: Rethinking the Way We Treat Animals by Karen Dawn (New York: HarperCollins, 2008).

The Ultimate Vegan Guide by Erik Marcus (Santa Cruz, CA: Vegan.com, 2009). Free download available at www.vegan.com/ultimate-vegan-guide/.

FACTORY FARMING

Eating Animals by Jonathan Safran Foer (New York: Little, Brown and Co., 2009).

Meat Market: Animals, Ethics, and Money by Erik Marcus (Ithaca, NY: Brio Press, 2005).

www.veganoutreach.org/whyvegan/animals.html

www.peta.org/issues/Animals-Used-For-Food/default.aspx
www.mercyforanimals.org/
www.cok.net/

FOR VEGAN ATHLETES

Vegetarian Sports Nutrition: Food Choices and Eating Plans for Fitness and Performance by D. Enette Larson-Meyer (Champaign, IL: Human Kinetics, 2007).
www.veganhealth.org/articles/athletes

FOR CHILDREN AND TEENS

PETA's Vegan College Cookbook: 275 Easy, Cheap, and Delicious Recipes to Keep You Vegan at School by Starza Kolman and Marta Holmberg (Naperville, IL: Sourcebooks, 2009).
Student's Go Vegan Cookbook: Over 135 Quick, Easy, Cheap and Tasty Vegan Recipes by Carole Raymond (New York: Three Rivers Press, 2006).
Vegan Lunch Box: 130 Amazing, Animal-Free Lunches Kids and Grown-Ups Will Love! by Jennifer McCann (Cambridge, MA: Da Capo Press, 2008).

BLOGS FOR VEGAN FAMILIES

www.tofu-n-sproutz.blogspot.com/
www.vegaloca.blogspot.com/
www.vegandad.blogspot.com/
www.yourveganmom.com/

GENERAL VEGAN COOKBOOKS

1000 Vegan Recipes by Robin Robertson (Hoboken, NJ: John Wiley and Sons, 2009).
The Conscious Cook: Delicious Meatless Recipes that Will Change the Way You Eat by Tal Ronnen (New York: HarperCollins, 2009).
The New Soy Cookbook by Lorna Sass (San Francisco: Chronicle Books, 1998).

Quick and Easy Vegan Comfort Food by Alicia C. Simpson (New York: The Experiment, 2009).

The Saucy Vegetarian by Joanne Stepaniak (Summertown, TN: Book Publishing Co., 2000).

Tofu Cookery, 25th anniversary ed., by Louise Hagler (Summertown, TN: Book Publishing Co., 2008).

The Ultimate Uncheese Cookbook: Delicious Dairy-Free Cheeses and Classic "Uncheese" Dishes by Joanne Stepaniak (Summertown, TN: Book Publishing Co., 1994).

Vegan Brunch: Homestyle Recipes Worth Waking Up For by Isa Chandra Moskowitz (Cambridge, MA: Da Capo Press, 2009).

Veganomicon: The Ultimate Vegan Cookbook by Isa Chandra Moskowitz and Terry Hope Romero (New York: Marlowe and Company, 2007).

Vegan on the Cheap: Great Recipes and Simple Strategies that Save You Time and Money by Robin Robertson (Hoboken, NJ: John Wiley and Sons, 2010).

Vegan Yum Yum: Decadent (But Doable) Animal-Free Recipes for Entertaining and Everyday by Lauren Ulm (Deerfield Beach, FL: Health Communications, 2009).

COOKBOOKS FOR VEGAN BAKING AND DESSERTS

More Great Good Dairy-Free Desserts Naturally by Fran Costigan (Summertown, TN: Book Publishing Co., 2006).

The Joy of Vegan Baking by Colleen Patrick-Goudreau (Beverly, MA: Quayside Publishing, 2007).

Sweet Utopia: Simply Stunning Vegan Desserts by Sharon Valencik (Summertown, TN: Book Publishing Co., 2009).

Vegan Cookies Take Over Your Cookie Jar by Isa Chandra Moskowitz and Terry Hope Romero (Cambridge, MA: Da Capo Press, 2009).

Vegan Cupcakes Take Over the World by Isa Chandra Moskowitz and Terry Hope Romero (Cambridge, MA: Da Capo Press, 2006).

RESOURCES FOR SPECIAL CIRCUMSTANCES

www.allergyfreeshop.com

The Everything Vegan Pregnancy Book by Reed Mangels (Avon, MA: Adams Media, 2011).

Food Allergy Survival Guide by Vesanto Melina, Jo Stepaniak, and Dina
   Aronson (Summertown, TN: Healthy Living Publications, 2004).
The Vegetarian Diet for Kidney Disease Treatment by Joan Brookhyser Hogan
   (Laguna Beach, CA: Basic Health Publications, 2009).

RECOMMENDED VEGAN FOOD AND COOKING BLOGS

www.meettheshannons.net/p/betty-crocker-project.html (This is the Betty
   Crocker Project, which is devoted to veganizing every recipe in the 1950
   Betty Crocker Picture Cookbook).
www.veganfeastkitchen.blogspot.com/
www.sharonsweets.wordpress.com/
www.elizaveganpage.blogspot.com/
www.veganeatsandtreats.blogspot.com/
www.veganinamericasdairyland.com/
www.vegangoodthings.blogspot.com/

A QUICK GUIDE TO COOKING GRAINS, BEANS, AND VEGETABLES

Whether or not you like to cook, it's good to know a few basics for preparing beans, grains, and vegetables.

COOKING DRIED BEANS

Regardless of the type of beans you cook, the technique is the same; it's just the time that varies. Contrary to popular opinion, you don't need to soak your beans. It tends to make them more easily digested, but vegan chef Bryanna Clark Grogan points out that Mexican cooks don't soak their beans. In fact, she says that Old World beans—like chickpeas and soybeans—cook better when soaked while all other beans—like pintos and black beans—can easily be cooked without soaking. Lentils and split peas should never be soaked.

Here are the steps to cooking dried beans:

1. Rinse the beans in a colander.
2. If you are soaking the beans, place them in a large pot or bowl with three cups of water for every cup of dried beans (that works out to about six cups of water for a pound of dried beans).
3. Allow beans to soak for at least four hours in the refrigerator. You can soak them for longer, and it's easy to put them to soak before going to bed at night and cook them for dinner the next evening.
4. Drain and rinse the beans.

5. Place the beans in a large pot and add either vegetable broth (for very flavorful beans) or plain salted water. Add three cups of liquid for every cup of dried beans that were soaked. Bring the liquid to a boil, reduce to a simmer, and cook until beans are tender—about one to two hours depending on the type of bean.

Cooked beans will keep in the refrigerator for four to five days. You can also freeze them. This will change their texture and taste slightly, but it's a good way to make sure you always have beans on hand. Cooked beans will keep in the freezer for about six months.

Cooking Times for Beans

These cooking times are ballpark figures. Actual cooking time depends on the size of the bean and its freshness. (The beans that have been stored in your pantry for a couple of years will take much longer to cook!)

Type of bean	Cooking time for soaked beans	Cooking time for unsoaked beans
Baby lima beans	45 to 60 minutes	
Black beans	1 to 1 ½ hours	2 ¼ to 2 ½ hours
Black-eyed peas	30 to 45 minutes	1 ½ to 1 ¾ hours
Cannellini beans	1 to 1 ¼ hours	1 ½ to 1 ¾ hours
Chickpeas	1 ½ to 2 hours	2 ½ to 3 hours
Great northern beans	1 to 1 ¼ hours	1 ½ to 1 ¾ hours
Navy beans	1 to 1 ¼ hours	1 ½ to 1 ¾ hours
Pinto beans	1 to 1 ¼ hours	1 ½ to 1 ¾ hours
Kidney beans	1 to 1 ¼ hours	1 ½ to 1 ¾ hours
Lentils	30 to 40 minutes	

GRAINS

Grains are at the center of life throughout the world, and they have been since the beginning of agriculture—about 12,000 years ago. It's fun to explore different grains, especially those used in different cultures.

Rice is the most popular grain in the world. Brown rice is much more healthful than white—but for traditional ethnic dishes, feel free to enjoy white rice on occasion if it fits the dish. Some favorites are basmati rice for Indian dishes, jasmine rice or sticky rice for Thai cuisine, or Arborio rice for creamy Italian risotto.

Other good grains to explore are barley, an old-fashioned favorite for soups; quinoa, which has been a staple in the Andes Mountains for centuries; fast-cooking couscous for Mediterranean salads; and chewy wheat berries for hearty winter stews.

Cooking Grains

Many cooks use rice cookers for all types of grains. They automatically shut off when cooking is complete and keep the food warm. If you cook a lot of grains, a rice cooker might be a worthwhile investment.

These instructions are for cooking grains on the stovetop. The time needed for different grains varies, but the technique is the same. For each cup of dry grain, bring two cups of water (or broth) to a boil. Add the grain, cover the pot with a lid, and lower the heat. Let simmer until all of the liquid is absorbed and the grain is tender. Here are cooking times for different grains:

Grain	Cooking Time
Barley, hulled	1 ½ hours
Barley, pearled	50 minutes
Couscous	5 minutes
Quinoa*	15 minutes
Rice, white	20 minutes
Rice, brown	40 minutes
Wheat berries	2 hours

*Always give quinoa a thorough rinse before cooking. It is coated with a natural insecticide that won't hurt you, but can give your dish a sort of soapy flavor.

VEGETABLES

Most of the work in preparing vegetables involves washing, peeling, paring, and chopping. If you don't have time for fresh vegetables, frozen or even canned are perfectly healthy choices. Check the produce section of your supermarket for packages of veggies that have already been washed and chopped. You'll find baby peeled carrots, precut and washed broccoli and cauliflower florets, broccoli slaw (shredded broccoli stalks—great for stir-fries), salad mixes, cabbage shredded for coleslaw, washed spinach, and more.

When it comes to cooking fresh veggies, the same technique works well for almost all vegetables: steaming followed by a quick sauté. (The exception is leafy greens: They require their own cooking technique, which is described below.) Here are the steps for cooking just about any type of vegetable:

1. Clean vegetables and remove any inedible portions.
2. Cut into bite-size pieces.
3. Place a steamer basket in a large, deep pan filled with about an inch of water. Heat the water to boiling, place the veggies in the basket, cover and steam until they reach desired tenderness.
4. Lift the steamer basket out of the pot (use a pot holder) and pour off the water. You can eat them as is, or do a quick sauté to bring out their flavor.
5. Add a tablespoon or two of olive oil to the pot and add the veggies. Add any seasonings you like and cook for a minute or so.

Cooking Leafy Greens

Steaming vegetables is one of the most healthful ways to cook them, but it doesn't work for leafy greens like collards, kale, mustard, and turnip greens. Here is a good technique from the cookbook *Greens Glorious Greens*.

1. Tear the greens into bite-size pieces. You can include the stems or not—it's up to you.
2. Plunge the greens into a big bowl of cold water and swish them around to clean. Drain the water. Repeat a couple of times to remove the grit that sometimes clings to the leaves.
3. While cleaning the greens, bring about two cups of water per pound of greens to boil in a large pot. Add the greens. Cover and boil for eight to ten minutes. Drain the greens.

As we directed for the vegetables above, you can give the greens a quick sauté in a bit of olive oil and season them. Here are tasty flavoring ideas for leafy greens:

Sauté onions with a clove of minced garlic and a pinch of cinnamon. Stir in the cooked greens.

Sauté chopped onions and garlic in olive oil. Add ¼ teaspoon of ground cayenne (more or less to taste) and salt and black pepper. Add a pound of cooked greens.

If you find that the taste of fresh greens is too strong at first, try tempering them with something creamy and bland. Puree silken tofu and mix into the greens with salt and pepper. Or mix in leftover mashed potatoes and soymilk.

METRIC CONVERSION CHART

- The recipes in this book have not been tested with metric measurements, so some variations might occur.
- Remember that the weight of dry ingredients varies according to the volume or density factor: 1 cup of flour weighs far less than 1 cup of sugar, and 1 tablespoon doesn't necessarily hold 3 teaspoons.

General Formulas for Metric Conversion

Ounces to grams	→	ounces × 28.35 = grams
Grams to ounces	→	grams × 0.035 = ounces
Pounds to grams	→	pounds × 453.5 = grams
Pounds to kilograms	→	pounds × 0.45 = kilograms
Cups to liters	→	cups × 0.24 = liters
Fahrenheit to Celsius	→	(°F − 32) × 5 ÷ 9 = °C
Celsius to Fahrenheit	→	(°C × 9) ÷ 5 + 32 = °F

Linear Measurements

½ inch	=	1½ cm
1 inch	=	2½ cm
6 inches	=	15 cm
8 inches	=	20 cm
10 inches	=	25 cm
12 inches	=	30 cm
20 inches	=	50 cm

Volume (Dry) Measurements

¼ teaspoon = 1 milliliter
½ teaspoon = 2 milliliters
¾ teaspoon = 4 milliliters
1 teaspoon = 5 milliliters
1 tablespoon = 15 milliliters
¼ cup = 59 milliliters
⅓ cup = 79 milliliters
½ cup = 118 milliliters
⅔ cup = 158 milliliters
¾ cup = 177 milliliters
1 cup = 225 milliliters
4 cups or 1 quart = 1 liter
½ gallon = 2 liters
1 gallon = 4 liters

Volume (Liquid) Measurements

1 teaspoon = ⅙ fluid ounce = 5 milliliters
1 tablespoon = ½ fluid ounce = 15 milliliters
2 tablespoons = 1 fluid ounce = 30 milliliters
¼ cup = 2 fluid ounces = 60 milliliters
⅓ cup = 2⅔ fluid ounces = 79 milliliters
½ cup = 4 fluid ounces = 118 milliliters
1 cup or ½ pint = 8 fluid ounces = 250 milliliters
2 cups or 1 pint = 16 fluid ounces = 500 milliliters
4 cups or 1 quart = 32 fluid ounces = 1,000 milliliters
1 gallon = 4 liters

Oven Temperature Equivalents, Fahrenheit (F) and Celsius (C)

100°F = 38°C
200°F = 95°C
250°F = 120°C
300°F = 150°C
350°F = 180°C
400°F = 205°C
450°F = 230°C

Weight (Mass) Measurements

1 ounce = 30 grams
2 ounces = 55 grams
3 ounces = 85 grams
4 ounces = ¼ pound = 125 grams
8 ounces = ½ pound = 240 grams
12 ounces = ¾ pound = 375 grams
16 ounces = 1 pound = 454 grams

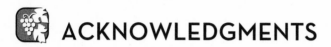 # ACKNOWLEDGMENTS

FROM JACK AND GINNY:

Thank you to our team of experts at Da Capo Press—editor Renée Sedliar, editorial assistant Erica Truxler, project editor Collin Tracy, designer Trish Wilkinson, and copyeditor Nancy King—for their skillful editing, patient guidance, and enthusiasm for this project. We couldn't imagine a better publishing experience and are grateful to our agent, Angela Miller, for believing in this book and helping us find the perfect home for it.

FROM JACK:

Thank you to Matt Ball, Anne Green, and the rest of Vegan Outreach, who have stood by my nutrition recommendations and writings when my perspective has not always been the most popular.

Ginny Messina was my first mentor in vegan nutrition, and I am honored to have written a book with her. Dr. Michael Greger, Dr. Stephen Walsh, Dr. Paul Appleby, Dr. Reed Mangels, Dr. Mark Messina, Tom Billings, and Brenda Davis have all helped me with research and understanding nutrition. Thank you!

My brother Eric was the first person in my family to boycott the products of factory farms, and I am thankful for all the support and friendship he has given me. I greatly look forward to meeting his and his wife, Thea's, baby, Dylan, who is due to arrive right before this book is published. My brother Todd is one of my best friends, and I am thankful that while our roots are 2,000 miles away in Cincinnati, only the San Francisco Bay separates us now.

My parents, Jack and Sylvia Norris, have given me their unconditional love and support and have always put my happiness ahead of theirs. You inspire me with your zest for life and genuine kindness towards everyone you meet!

Thank you to Eric Marcus for all the valuable help you have given me with my blog and all you do to promote compassion to animals.

Thank you to my friends who work so hard on behalf of farmed animals. You are moving mountains:

Jon Camp, Joe Espinosa, Eugene Khtoryansky, Casey Constable, Vic Sjodin, Stewart Solomon, Brian Grupe, Nikki Benoit, Eileen Botti, Rick Hershey, Fred Tyler, Phil Letten, Rob Gilbride and Eleni Vlachos, Leslie Patterson, Jeff Boghosian and Dawn R, Star Sevadar, Nick and Anna Lesiecki, Nick Cooney, Aaron Ross and Kate St. John, Lana Smithson, Barbara Bear, Amanda Schemkes, Darina Smith, Lauren Panos, Steve Kaufman, John and Fany Borger, Michele and Chris Christensen, Mark and Kristie Middleton, Keyur and Shilpa Shah, Vicky and Charlie Talbert, Dan Phillips, Rebecca and Ariel Nessel, Dave Bemel, Bruce Friedrich and Alka Chandna, Paul Shapiro, Erica Meier, Josh Balk, lauren Ornelas, Kim Sturla, Eugene Patrick, Kath Rogers and Bryan Peas, Jodi Chemes, Armaiti May, Lisa Shapiro, Gene Baur, Jason Matheny, and Nathan Runkle and all the amazing MFA activists.

To my good friends Mark Foy and Eric Roberts, I'm so glad you ended up in the Bay Area! And to the rest of the local heroes: Tammy Lee and Chris James, Shani Campbell, Michelle Cehn and Dan Miller, Henry Chen, and the rest of the Oakland PETA crew. To my out-of-towner friends Tony Hannemann, Clint Buttler and Ruby Mani, Charlotte Markee, Monica Engebretson and Philip Wright, and Phil Murray and Shari Kalina.

Thank you to Ingrid Newkirk of PETA and to Peter Singer, whose writings and activism initially inspired me to get involved in animal protection. And to my early animal activist mentors: Tim and Sue Huesken, Jayn and Tom Meinhardt, and Alex Hershaft.

To Kevin Gallagher: Thank you for your friendship, your support, and your insanity. It has been a pleasure, sir.

To my wife, Alex: Your love for animals shines. Thank you for believing in me.

FROM GINNY:

In my twenty-plus years as a vegan dietitian, I've been honored to work with some of the most knowledgeable and dedicated vegan nutrition professionals. Thank you especially to Dr. Reed Mangels for her friendship and collaboration over the years and for reviewing parts of this book. She and dietitians Dr. Suzanne Havala-Hobbs, Dr. Winston Craig, Vesanto Melina, Brenda Davis, and the late Cyndi Reeser have been true pioneers who established vegetarianism as an area of practice in the field of nutrition. It is a privilege to know these extraordinary people as colleagues and friends. And a special thank-you to Jack Norris for his dedication to sharing the best and most accurate nutrition information and for inviting me to write this book with him.

Charles Stahler and Debra Wasserman of the Vegetarian Resource Group earned my ongoing appreciation twenty years ago, when they gave me an opportunity to develop my skills as a vegan dietitian and invited me into their community of activists and educators.

Erik Marcus is committed to finding the absolute best ways to advocate for animals and is a daily source of inspiration and information. I'm grateful for his work, his friendship and his enthusiasm for this book.

Thank you to Matt Ball and Anne Green of Vegan Outreach for their support of my work and for the wisdom and insight they bring to animal advocacy. They are among my personal heroes.

Dr. Neal Barnard, president of the Physicians Committee for Responsible Medicine, gave me my first job as a vegan dietitian and taught me a great deal about writing and advocacy. My work with Neal and PCRM opened many doors and put me on a professional path I would never have imagined. I am forever grateful.

My former agent Patti Breitman championed this book from the start and worked hard to help us find an agent. Her efforts to make sure that vegan books find publishers has had a far-reaching impact on animal lives.

Dr. Michael Klaper is the best kind of physician—one who uses his extensive medical knowledge to advocate for compassionate food choices and to protect the health of vegans. He has been a role model for as long as I've worked in this field.

Dustin Rhodes and Lee Hall of Friends of Animals, and Leah McKelvie are among the kindest people I know. They encourage respect and helpfulness within a community encompassing divergent views, and I've learned a great deal from all of them.

Louise Holton, president of Alley Cat Rescue, has long been my model for compassion. She has done more to help feral cats than any person in the world, and she continues to be an advocate for farm animals and veganism as well.

To my buddies at goodreads.com, especially Lisa Herzstein: Thank you for sharing my passions for the most important things in life—animals and books—and for proving that online social networking can produce meaningful and gratifying connections.

My friend Kate Schumann has collaborated with me on projects beginning with our vegan cookbook-writing days at PCRM through our work on behalf of companion animals in Port Townsend. She is not only a wonderful friend but also a brilliant cook, gardener, educator, and designer, and she shares her knowledge generously. She also belongs to a group of the hardest working women I know—the board of directors of Olympic Mountain Pet Pals: Phyllis Becker, Pam Gray, Robin Hake, Pam Kolacy, Carolynn Moody, Donna Regester, Erica Springstead, Marsha Wiener, and Randi Winter. My experience as part of this organization has been an amazing education in grassroots advocacy and fund-raising.

And a special thank-you to Dr. Ginny Johnson for her work with local rescue groups, her devoted care of my own family of cats, and her commitment to veganism and justice for all animals. There is not a more generous animal advocate anywhere.

My fourth-grade teacher made it a point to instill confidence in the shyest kid in class by praising my reports and essays and encouraging me to work hard on my writing skills. I listened to your advice, Mrs. Kellogg, and have never forgotten your kindness.

Thank you to my dear family and friends, whose love and support are blessings beyond measure: My brothers, Bill Kisch and Steve Kisch; sisters-in-law, Irma Kisch, Agnes Kisch, and Pat Gordon; beautiful nieces, Sarah Gordon, Christen Kisch, and Heather Kisch; wonderful nephews, Noah Gordon, Bogart Kisch, Chris Kisch, and dear little Reid Ellie Kisch. And thank you to Debbi Zabel, Joan Petrokofsky, Lynn Myhal Zornetzer, and Diana Longo for being my BFFs and filling my life with fun, laughter, comfort, and love. And to Paige Pettit, the world's best cat nanny, and Kathy Ostgaard for all those exhausting (but fun) garage sale fund-raisers.

To my mom and dad, Willie Schrenk Kisch and Bill Kisch, who are temporarily gone from my sight but always in my heart. A list of their gifts to me could fill a whole book.

I don't know how anyone gets any work done unless they have at least three cats snoozing on their desk. Thank you to the beloved kitties who kept me company during the long hours spent writing this book and to all the ferals, fosters, and spoiled house cats who have graced my life and home over the years.

Finally, I am blessed and grateful every day to be married to Mark Messina. He holds me accountable for every single thing I say about nutrition, makes me laugh, and (almost) never complains when I bring home stray cats.

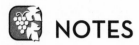 NOTES

INTRODUCTION: GOING VEGAN FOR LIFE

1. W. J. Craig and A. R. Mangels, "Position of the American Dietetic Association: Vegetarian Diets," *Journal of the American Dietetic Association* 109, no. 7 (2009): 1266–82.

CHAPTER 1: UNDERSTANDING VEGAN NUTRIENT NEEDS

1. R. Elango, M. A. Humayun, R. O. Ball, and P. B. Pencharz, "Evidence that Protein Requirements Have Been Significantly Underestimated," *Current Opinion in Clinical Nutrition & Metabolic Care* 13, no. 1 (2010): 52–57.

2. R. Mangels, V. Messina, and M. Messina, *The Dietitian's Guide to Vegetarian Diets*, 3rd ed. (Sudbury, MA: Jones and Bartlett, 2010), 530–54.

3. G. K. Davey, E. A. Spencer, P. N. Appleby, N. E. Allen, K. H. Knox, and T. J. Key, "EPIC-Oxford: Lifestyle Characteristics and Nutrient Intakes in a Cohort of 33,883 Meat-eaters and 31,546 Non-meat-eaters in the UK," *Public Health Nutrition* 6, no. 3 (2003): 259–69.

4. B. J. Abelow, T. R. Holford, and K. L. Insogna, "Cross-Cultural Association between Dietary Animal Protein and Hip Fracture: A Hypothesis." *Calcified Tissue International* 50, no. 1 (1992): 14–18.

CHAPTER 2: PROTEIN FROM PLANTS

1. V. R. Young and P. L. Pellett, "Plant Proteins in Relation to Human Protein and Amino Acid Nutrition," *American Journal of Clinical Nutrition* 59, suppl. no. 5 (1994): S1203–S1212.

2. F. M. Lappé, *Diet for a Small Planet* (New York: Ballantine, 1971), 72–94.

3. M. F. Fuller and P. J. Reeds, "Nitrogen Cycling in the Gut," *Annual Review of Nutrition* 18 (1998): 385–411.

4. G. Sarwar, "Digestibility of Protein and Bioavailability of Amino Acids in Foods: Effects on Protein Quality Assessment," *World Review of Nutrition and Dietetics* 54 (1987): 26–70.

5. R. Elango, M. A. Humayun, R. O. Ball, and P. B. Pencharz, "Evidence that Protein Requirements Have Been Significantly Underestimated," *Current Opinion in Clinical Nutrition & Metabolic Care* 13, no. 1 (2010): 52–57.

6. C. Hudson, S. Hudson, and J. MacKenzie, "Protein-Source Tryptophan as an Efficacious Treatment for Social Anxiety Disorder: A Pilot Study," *Canadian Journal of Physiology and Pharmacology* 85, no. 9 (2007): 928–32.

CHAPTER 3: VITAMIN B12: THE GORILLA IN THE ROOM

1. H. Van den Berg, P. C. Dagnelie, and W. A. Van Staveren. "Vitamin B12 and Seaweed," *Lancet* 1 (1988): 242–43.

2. R. Carmel, D. S. Karnaze, and J. M. Weiner, "Neurologic Abnormalities in Cobalamin Deficiency are Associated with Higher Cobalamin 'Analogue' Values than are Hematologic Abnormalities," *Journal of Laboratory and Clinical Medicine* 111, no. 1 (1988): 57–62.

3. K. Yamada, Y. Yamada, M. Fukuda, S. Yamada. "Bioavailability of Dried Asa-Kusanori (porphyra tenera) as a Source of Cobalamin (Vitamin B12)," *International Journal for Vitamin and Nutrition Research* 69, no. 6 (1999): 412–8.

4. A. Mozafar and J. J. Oertli, "Uptake of a Microbially-Produced Vitamin (B12) by Soybean Roots," *Plant Soil* 139 (1992): 23–30.

5. W. J. Craig and A. R. Mangels, "Position of the American Dietetic Association: Vegetarian Diets," *Journal of the American Dietetic Association* 109, no. 7 (2009): 1266–82.

6. C. Antoniades, A. S. Antonopoulos, D. Tousoulis, K. Marinou, and C. Stefanadis, "Homocysteine and Coronary Atherosclerosis: From Folate Fortification to the Recent Clinical Trials," *European Heart Journal* 30, no. 1 (2009): 6–15.

7. F. Van Dam, W. A. Van Gool, "Hyperhomocysteinemia and Alzheimer's Disease: A Systematic Review," *Archives of Gerontology and Geriatrics* 48 (2009): 425–30.

8. A. M. Molloy, P. N. Kirke, J. F. Troendle, et al., "Maternal Vitamin B12 Status and Risk of Neural Tube Defects in a Population with High Neural Tube Defect Prevalence and No Folic Acid Fortification," *Pediatrics* 123, no. 3 (2009): 917–23.

9. Jack Norris, "Mild B12 Deficiency–Elevated Homocysteine," www.vegan health.org/b12/hcy.

10. L. H. Allen, "How Common Is Vitamin B-12 Deficiency?" *American Journal of Clinical Nutrition* 89, no. 2 (2009): S693–S696.

11. B. D. Hokin and T. Butler, "Cyanocobalamin (Vitamin B-12) Status in Seventh-day Adventist Ministers in Australia," *American Journal of Clinical Nutrition* 70, suppl. no. 3 (1999): S576–S578.

12. Robert Mason, "Afarensis May Have Eaten Meat: So What?" August 4, 2010, http://paleovegan.blogspot.com/2010/08/afarensis-may-have-used-stone-tools-so.html.

13. Tom Billings, "Comparative Anatomy and Physiology Brought Up to Date," http://www.beyondveg.com/billings-t/comp-anat/comp-anat-9e.shtml.

CHAPTER 4: CALCIUM, VITAMIN D, AND BONE HEALTH

1. S. B. Eaton and D. A. Nelson, "Calcium in Evolutionary Perspective," *American Journal of Clinical Nutrition* 54, suppl. no. 1 (1991): S281–S287.

2. R. Mangels, V. Messina, and M. Messina, *The Dietitian's Guide to Vegetarian Diets*, 3rd ed. (Sudbury, MA: Jones and Bartlett, 2010), 520–29.

3. D. Feskanich, W. C. Willett, M. J. Stampfer, and G. A. Colditz, "Milk, Dietary Calcium, and Bone Fractures in Women: A 12-Year Prospective Study," *American Journal of Public Health* 87, no. 6 (1997): 992–97.

4. H. A. Bischoff-Ferrari, B. Dawson-Hughes, J. A. Baron, et al., "Calcium Intake and Hip Fracture Risk in Men and Women: A Meta-Analysis of Prospective Cohort Studies and Randomized Controlled Trials," *American Journal of Clinical Nutrition* 86, no. 6 (2007): 1780–90.

5. B. M. Tang, G. D. Eslick, C. Nowson, C. Smith, and A. Bensoussan, "Use of Calcium or Calcium in Combination with Vitamin D Supplementation to Prevent Fractures and Bone Loss in People Aged 50 Years and Older: A Meta-Analysis," *Lancet* 370, no. 9588 (2007): 657–66.

6. B. J. Abelow, T. R. Holford, and K. L. Insogna, "Cross-Cultural Association between Dietary Animal Protein and Hip Fracture: A Hypothesis," *Calcified Tissue International* 50, no. 1 (1992): 14–18.

7. R. J. Wetzsteon, J. M. Hughes, B. C. Kaufman, et al., "Ethnic Differences in Bone Geometry and Strength Are Apparent in Childhood," *Bone* 44, no. 5 (2009): 970–75.

8. K. G. Faulkner, S. R. Cummings, D. Black, L. Palermo, C. C. Gluer, and H. K. Genant, "Simple Measurement of Femoral Geometry Predicts Hip Fracture: The Study of Osteoporotic Fractures," *Journal of Bone and Mineral Research* 8, no. 10 (1993): 1211–17.

9. M. Russell-Aulet, J. Wang, J. C. Thornton, E. W. Colt, and R. N. Pierson, Jr., "Bone Mineral Density and Mass in a Cross-Sectional Study of White

and Asian Women," *Journal of Bone and Mineral Research* 8, no. 5 (1993): 575–82.

10. H. Spencer, L. Kramer, M. DeBartolo, C. Norris, and D. Osis, "Further Studies of the Effect of a High-Protein Diet as Meat on Calcium Metabolism," *American Journal of Clinical Nutrition* 37, no. 6 (1983): 924–29.

11. J. E. Kerstetter, K. O. O'Brien, and K. L. Insogna, "Dietary Protein Affects Intestinal Calcium Absorption," *American Journal of Clinical Nutrition* 68, no. 4 (1998): 859–65.

12. J. E. Kerstetter, A. C. Looker, and K. L. Insogna, "Low Dietary Protein and Low Bone Density," *Calcified Tissue International* 66, no. 4 (2000): 313.

13. M. A. Schurch, R. Rizzoli, D. Slosman, L. Vadas, P. Vergnaud, and J. P. Bonjour, "Protein Supplements Increase Serum Insulin-like Growth Factor-I Levels and Attenuate Proximal Femur Bone Loss in Patients with Recent Hip Fracture: A Randomized, Double-blind, Placebo-controlled Trial," *Annals of Internal Medicine* 128, no. 10 (1998): 801–09.

14. Ibid.

15. P. Appleby, A. Roddam, N. Allen, and T. Key, "Comparative Fracture Risk in Vegetarians and Nonvegetarians in EPIC-Oxford," *European Journal of Clinical Nutrition* 61, no. 12 (2007): 1400–06.

16. C. M. Weaver and K. L. Plawecki, "Dietary Calcium: Adequacy of a Vegetarian Diet," *American Journal of Clinical Nutrition* 59, suppl. no. 5 (1994): S1238–S1241.

17. G. Schwalfenberg, "Not Enough Vitamin D: Health Consequences for Canadians," *Canadian Family Physician* 53, no. 5 (2007): 841–54.

18. L. A. Armas, B. W. Hollis, and R. P. Heaney, "Vitamin D2 is Much Less Effective than Vitamin D3 in Humans," *Journal of Clinical Endocrinology and Metabolism* 89, no. 11 (2004): 5387–91.

19. M. F. Holick, R. M. Biancuzzo, T. C. Chen, E. K. Klein, A. Young, D. Bibuld, R. Reitz, W. Salameh, A. Ameri, and A. D. Tannenbaum, "Vitamin D2 Is as Effective as Vitamin D3 in Maintaining Circulating Concentrations of 25-Hydroxyvitamin D," *Journal of Clinical Endocrinology and Metabolism* 93, no. 3 (2008): 677–81.

20. T. A. Outila, M. U. Karkkainen, R. H. Seppanen, and C. J. Lamberg-Allardt, "Dietary Intake of Vitamin D in Premenopausal, Healthy Vegans Was Insufficient to Maintain Concentrations of Serum 25-Hydroxyvitamin D and Intact Parathyroid Hormone within Normal Ranges During the Winter in Finland," *Journal of the American Dietetic Association* 100, no. 4 (2000): 434–41.

21. B. L. Specker, B. Valanis, V. Hertzberg, N. Edwards, and R. C. Tsang, "Sunshine Exposure and Serum 25-Hydroxyvitamin D Concentrations in Exclusively Breast-fed Infants," *Journal of Pediatrics* 107, no. 3 (1985): 372–76.

22. T. L. Clemens, J. S. Adams, S. L. Henderson, and M. F. Holick, "Increased Skin Pigment Reduces the Capacity of Skin to Synthesise Vitamin D3," *Lancet* 1, no. 8263 (1982): 74–76.

23. M. F. Holick, L. Y. Matsuoka, and J. Wortsman, "Age, Vitamin D, and Solar Ultraviolet," *Lancet* 2, no. 8671 (1989): 1104–05.

CHAPTER 5: FATS: MAKING THE BEST CHOICES

1. U. J. Jung, C. Torrejon, A. P. Tighe, and R. J. Deckelbaum, "N-3 Fatty Acids and Cardiovascular Disease: Mechanisms Underlying Beneficial Effects," *American Journal of Clinical Nutrition* 87, no. 6 (2008): S2003–S2009.

2. M. C. Morris, D. A. Evans, J. L. Bienias, et al., "Consumption of Fish and N-3 Fatty Acids and Risk of Incident Alzheimer's Disease," *Archives of Neurology* 60, no. 7 (2003): 940–46.

3. P. Y. Lin and K. P. Su, "A Meta-analytic Review of Double-Blind, Placebo-Controlled Trials of Antidepressant Efficacy of Omega-3 Fatty Acids," *Journal of Clinical Psychiatry* 68, no. 7 (2007): 1056–61.

4. N. Mann, Y. Pirotta, S. O'Connell, D. Li, F. Kelly, and A. Sinclair, "Fatty Acid Composition of Habitual Omnivore and Vegetarian Diets," *Lipids* 41, no. 7 (2006): 637–46.

5. D. Mezzano, X. Munoz, C. Martinez, et al., "Vegetarians and Cardiovascular Risk Factors: Hemostasis, Inflammatory Markers and Plasma Homocysteine," *Journal of Thrombosis and Haemostasis* 81, no. 6 (1999): 913–17.

6. D. Mezzano, K. Kosiel, C. Martínez, A. Cuevas, O. Panes, E. Aranda, P. Strobel, D. D. Pérez, J. Pereira, J. Rozowski, and F. Leighton, "Cardiovascular Risk Factors in Vegetarians: Normalization of Hyperhomocysteinemia with Vitamin B12 and Reduction of Platelet Aggregation with N-3 Fatty Acids," *Thrombosis Research* 100, no. 3 (2000): 153–60.

7. T. A. Sanders and F. Roshanai, "Platelet Phospholipid Fatty Acid Composition and Function in Vegans Compared with Age-and Sex-Matched Omnivore Controls," *European Journal of Clinical Nutrition* 46, no. 11 (1992): 823–31.

8. T. J. Key, G. E. Fraser, M. Thorogood, et al., "Mortality in Vegetarians and Nonvegetarians: Detailed Findings from a Collaborative Analysis of 5 Prospective Studies," *American Journal of Clinical Nutrition* 70, suppl. no. 3 (1999): S516–S524.

9. R. Mangels, V. Messina, and M. Messina, *The Dietitian's Guide to Vegetarian Diets*, 3rd ed. (Sudbury, MA: Jones and Bartlett, 2010), 517–19.

10. E. Cho, S. Hung, W. C. Willett, et al., "Prospective Study of Dietary Fat and the Risk of Age-Related Macular Degeneration," *American Journal of Clinical Nutrition* 73, no. 2 (2001): 209–18.

11. Z. Lloyd-Wright, R. Preston, R. Gray, et al., "Randomized Placebo Controlled Trial of a Daily Intake of 200 mg Docasahexanoic Acid in Vegans," abstract in *Proceedings of the Nutrition Society* 62 (2003): 42a.

12. J. A. Conquer and B. J. Holub, "Supplementation with an Algae Source of Docosahexaenoic Acid Increases (N-3) Fatty Acid Status and Alters Selected Risk Factors for Heart Disease in Vegetarian Subjects," *Journal of Nutrition* 126, no. 12 (1996): 3032–39.

13. Interim Summary of Conclusions and Dietary Recommendations on Total Fat and Fatty Acids: From the Joint FAO/WHO Expert Consultation on Fats and Fatty Acids in Human Nutrition, 10–14, November 2008, WHO, Geneva. http://www.who.int/nutrition/topics/FFA_summary_rec_conclusion.pdf.

CHAPTER 6: IRON, ZINC, IODINE, AND VITAMIN A: MAXIMIZING VEGAN SOURCES

1. R. Mangels, V. Messina, and M. Messina, *The Dietitian's Guide to Vegetarian Diets*, 3rd ed. (Sudbury, MA: Jones and Bartlett, 2010), 530–35.

2. Centers for Disease Control and Prevention, "Iron Deficiency—United States, 1999–2000," *Morbidity Mortality Weekly Report* 51 (2002): 897–99.

3. S. Seshadri, A. Shah, and S. Bhade, "Haematologic Response of Anaemic Preschool Children to Ascorbic Acid Supplementation," *Human Nutrition Applied Nutrition* 39, no. 2 (1985): 151–54.

4. Centers for Disease Control and Prevention, "Recommendations to Prevent and Control Iron Deficiency in the United States," *Morbidity Mortality Weekly Report* 47 (1998): 1–29.

5. J. D. Cook, S. A. Dassenko, and S. R. Lynch, "Assessment of the Role of Nonheme-Iron Availability in Iron Balance," *American Journal of Clinical Nutrition* 54, no. 4 (1991): 717–22.

6. D. H. Rushton, "Nutritional Factors and Hair Loss," *Clinical and Experimental Dermatology* 27, no. 5 (2002): 396–404.

7. Ibid.

8. P. N. Appleby, M. Thorogood, J. I. Mann, and T. J. Key, "The Oxford Vegetarian Study: An Overview," *American Journal of Clinical Nutrition* 70, suppl. no. 3 (1999): S525–S531.

9. S. L. Booth, K. L. Tucker, H. Chen, et al., "Dietary Vitamin K Intakes Are Associated with Hip Fracture but Not with Bone Mineral Density in Elderly Men and Women," *American Journal of Clinical Nutrition* 71, no. 5 (2000): 1201–08.

10. T. A. Sanders and F. Roshanai, "Platelet Phospholipid Fatty Acid Composition and Function in Vegans Compared with Age-and Sex-Matched Omnivore Controls," *European Journal of Clinical Nutrition* 46, no. 11 (1992): 823–31.

CHAPTER 9: A HEALTHY START:
VEGAN DIETS IN PREGNANCY AND BREAST-FEEDING

1. J. P. Carter, T. Furman, and H. R. Hutcheson, "Preeclampsia and Reproductive Performance in a Community of Vegans," *Southern Medical Journal* 80, no. 6 (1987): 692–97.

2. V. Lakin, P. Haggarty, D. R. Abramovich, et al., "Dietary Intake and Tissue Concentration of Fatty Acids in Omnivore, Vegetarian and Diabetic Pregnancy," *Prostaglandins Leukotrienes and Essential Fatty Acids* 59, no. 3 (1998): 209–20.

3. T. A. Sanders and S. Reddy, "The Influence of a Vegetarian Diet on the Fatty Acid Composition of Human Milk and the Essential Fatty Acid Status of the Infant," *Journal of Pediatrics* 120 (1992): S71–S77.

CHAPTER 10: RAISING VEGAN CHILDREN AND TEENS

1. Committee on Nutrition, American Academy of Pediatrics, Pediatric Nutrition Handbook, 6th ed. (Elk Grove, IL: American Academy of Pediatrics, 2009), 114–32.

2. A. R. Mangels and V. Messina, "Considerations in Planning Vegan Diets: Infants," *Journal of the American Dietetic Association* 101, no. 6 (2001): 670–77.

3. M. A. Mendez, M. S. Anthony, and L. Arab, "Soy-Based Formulae and Infant Growth and Development: A Review," *Journal of Nutrition* 132, no. 8 (2002): 2127–30.

4. V. Messina and A. R. Mangels, "Considerations in Planning Vegan Diets: Children," *Journal of the American Dietetic Association* 101, no. 6 (2001): 661–69.

5. K. C. Janelle and S. I. Barr, "Nutrient Intakes and Eating Behavior Scores of Vegetarian and Nonvegetarian Women," *Journal of the American Dietetic Association* 95, no. 2 (1995): 180–86, 189.

CHAPTER 11: VEGAN DIETS FOR PEOPLE OVER FIFTY

1. S. D. Krasinski, R. M. Russell, I. M. Samloff, et al., "Fundic Atrophic Gastritis in an Elderly Population: Effect on Hemoglobin and Several Serum Nutritional Indicators," *Journal of the American Geriatrics Society* 34, no. 11 (1986): 800–06.

2. B. M. Tang, G. D. Eslick, C. Nowson, C. Smith, and A. Bensoussan, "Use of Calcium or Calcium in Combination with Vitamin D Supplementation to Prevent Fractures and Bone Loss in People Aged 50 Years and Older: A Meta-analysis," *Lancet* 370, no. 9588 (2007): 657–66.

3. W. W. Campbell, "Dietary Protein Requirements of Older People: Is the RDA Adequate?" *Nutrition Today* 31 (1996): 192–97.

4. W. W. Campbell, "Synergistic Use of Higher-Protein Diets or Nutritional Supplements with Resistance Training to Counter Sarcopenia," *Nutrition Reviews* 65, no. 9 (2007): 416–22.

5. P. Glem, W. L. Beeson, and G. E. Fraser, "The Incidence of Dementia and Intake of Animal Products: Preliminary Findings from the Adventist Health Study," *Neuroepidemiology* 12 (1993): 28–36.

6. A. T. Hostmark, E. Lystad, O. D. Vellar, K. Hovi, and J. E. Berg, "Reduced Plasma Fibrinogen, Serum Peroxides, Lipids, and Apolipoproteins after a 3-Week Vegetarian Diet," *Plant Foods for Human Nutrition* 43, no. 1 (1993): 55–61.

CHAPTER 12: THE PLANT FOOD ADVANTAGE: HEALTH BENEFITS OF A VEGAN DIET

1. T. J. Key, G. E. Fraser, M. Thorogood, et al., "Mortality in Vegetarians and Nonvegetarians: Detailed Findings from a Collaborative Analysis of 5 Prospective Studies," *American Journal of Clinical Nutrition* 70, suppl. no. 3 (1999): S516–S524.

2. J. Norris, "Disease Markers of Vegetarians," http://www.veganhealth.org/articles/dxmarkers#totwest.

3. A. N. Donaldson, "The Relation of Protein Foods to Hypertension," *California and Western Medicine* 24 (1926): 328–31.

4. G. E. Fraser, "Vegetarian Diets: What Do We Know of Their Effects on Common Chronic Diseases?" *American Journal of Clinical Nutrition* 89, no. 5 (2009): S1607–S1612.

5. P. N. Appleby, G. K. Davey, and T. J. Key, "Hypertension and Blood Pressure among Meat Eaters, Fish Eaters, Vegetarians and Vegans in EPIC-Oxford," *Public Health Nutrition* 5, no. 5 (2002): 645–54.

6. S. Tonstad, T. Butler, R. Yan, and G. E. Fraser, "Type of Vegetarian Diet, Body Weight, and Prevalence of Type 2 Diabetes," *Diabetes Care* 32, no. 5 (2009): 791–96.

7. E. A. Spencer, P. N. Appleby, G. K. Davey, and T. J. Key, "Diet and Body Mass Index in 38000 EPIC-Oxford Meat-eaters, Fish-eaters, Vegetarians and Vegans," *International Journal of Obesity and Related Metabolic Disorders* 27, no. 6 (2003): 728–33.

CHAPTER 13: MANAGING WEIGHT, HEART DISEASE, AND DIABETES

1. A. Mente, L. De Koning, H. S. Shannon, and S. S. Anand, "A Systematic Review of the Evidence Supporting a Causal Link between Dietary Factors and Coronary Heart Disease," *Archives of Internal Medicine* 169, no. 7 (2009): 659–69.

2. P. W. Siri-Tarino, Q. Sun, F. B. Hu, and R. M. Krauss, "Meta-analysis of Prospective Cohort Studies Evaluating the Association of Saturated Fat with Cardiovascular Disease," *American Journal of Clinical Nutrition* 91, no. 3 (2010): 535–46.

3. F. B. Hu, "Diet and Lifestyle Influences on Risk of Coronary Heart Disease," *Current Atherosclerosis Reports* 11, no. 4 (2009): 257–63.

4. J. Sabate, K. Oda, and E. Ros, "Nut Consumption and Blood Lipid Levels: A Pooled Analysis of 25 Intervention Trials," *Archives of Internal Medicine* 170, no. 9 (2010): 821–27.

5. D. Ornish, S. E. Brown, L. W. Scherwitz, et al., "Can Lifestyle Changes Reverse Coronary Heart Disease? The Lifestyle Heart Trial," *Lancet* 336, no. 8708 (1990): 129–33.

6. N. D. Barnard, J. Cohen, D. J. Jenkins, et al., "A Low-fat Vegan Diet and a Conventional Diabetes Diet in the Treatment of Type 2 Diabetes: A Randomized, Controlled, 74-Week Clinical Trial," *American Journal of Clinical Nutrition* 89, no. 5 (2009): S1588–S1596.

7. Y. Cao, C. L. Pelkman, G. Zhao, S. M. Townsend, and P. M. Kris-Etherton, "Effects of Moderate (MF) versus Lower Fat (LF) Diets on Lipids and Lipoproteins: A Meta-analysis of Clinical Trials in Subjects with and without Diabetes," *Journal of Clinical Lipidology* 3 (2009): 19–32.

8. A. Garg, "High-Monounsaturated-Fat Diets for Patients with Diabetes Mellitus: A Meta-analysis," *American Journal of Clinical Nutrition* 67, suppl. no. 3 (1998): S577–S582.

9. W. C. Willett, "Will High-Carbohydrate/Low-Fat Diets Reduce the Risk of Coronary Heart Disease?" *Proceedings of the Society for Experimental Biology and Medicine* 225, no. 3 (2000): 187–90.

10. D. J. Gordon, J. L. Probstfield, R. J. Garrison, et al., "High-Density Lipoprotein Cholesterol and Cardiovascular Disease: Four Prospective American Studies," *Circulation* 79, no. 1 (1989): 8–15.

11. B. J. Arsenault, J. S. Rana, E. S. Stroes, et al., "Beyond Low-Density Lipoprotein Cholesterol: Respective Contributions of Non-high-density Lipoprotein Cholesterol Levels, Triglycerides, and the Total Cholesterol/High-Density Lipoprotein Cholesterol Ratio to Coronary Heart Disease Risk in Apparently Healthy Men and Women," *Journal of the American College of Cardiology* 55, no. 1 (2009): 35–41.

12. S. Cicerale, X. A. Conlan, A. J. Sinclair, and R. S. Keast, "Chemistry and Health of Olive Oil Phenolics," *Critical Reviews in Food Science and Nutrition* 49, no. 3 (2009): 218–36.

13. V. Remig, B. Franklin, S. Margolis, G. Kostas, T. Nece, and J. C. Street, "Trans Fats in America: A Review of Their Use, Consumption, Health Implications, and Regulation," *Journal of the American Dietetic Association* 110, no. 4 (2010): 585–92.

14. I. Abete, D. Parra, and J. A. Martinez, "Energy-Restricted Diets Based on a Distinct Food Selection Affecting the Glycemic Index Induce Different Weight Loss and Oxidative Response. *Clinical Nutrition* 27, no. 4 (2008): 545–51.

15. K. McManus, L. Antinoro, and F. Sacks, "A Randomized Controlled Trial of a Moderate-Fat, Low-Energy Diet Compared with a Low-Fat, Low-Energy Diet for Weight Loss in Overweight Adults," *International Journal of Obesity and Related Metabolic Disorders* 25, no. 10 (2001): 1503–11.

16. M. Bes-Rastrollo, N. M. Wedick, M. A. Martinez-Gonzalez, T. Y. Li, L. Sampson, and F. B. Hu, "Prospective Study of Nut Consumption, Long-Term Weight Change, and Obesity Risk in Women," *American Journal of Clinical Nutrition* 89, no. 6 (2009): 1913–19.

17. R. D. Mattes and M. L. Dreher, "Nuts and Healthy Body Weight Maintenance Mechanisms," *Asia Pacific Journal of Clinical Nutrition* 19, no. 1 (2010): 137–41.

CHAPTER 14: SPORTS NUTRITION

1. P. W. Lemon, M. A. Tarnopolsky, J. D. MacDougall, and S. A. Atkinson, "Protein Requirements and Muscle Mass/Strength Changes During Intensive Training in Novice Bodybuilders," *Journal of Applied Physiology* 73, no. 2 (1992): 767–75.

2. M. A. Tarnopolsky, J. D. MacDougall, and S. A. Atkinson, "Influence of Protein Intake and Training Status on Nitrogen Balance and Lean Body Mass," *Journal of Applied Physiology* 64, no. 1 (1988): 187–93.

3. N. R. Rodriguez, N. M. DiMarco, and S. Langley, "Position of the American Dietetic Association, Dietitians of Canada, and the American College of Sports Medicine: Nutrition and Athletic Performance," *Journal of the American Dietetic Association* 109, no. 3 (2009): 509–27.

4. Ibid.

5. P. Borrione, A. Spaccamiglio, R. A. Salvo, A. Mastrone, F. Fagnani, and F. Pigozzi, "Rhabdomyolysis in a Young Vegetarian Athlete," *American Journal of Physical Medicine and Rehabilitation* 88, no. 11 (2009): 951–54.

6. A. Shomrat, Y. Weinstein, and A. Katz, "Effect of Creatine Feeding on Maximal Exercise Performance in Vegetarians," *European Journal of Applied Physiology* 82, no. 4 (2000): 321–25.

7. C. J. Rebouche, E. P. Bosch, C. A. Chenard, K. J. Schabold, and S. E. Nelson, "Utilization of Dietary Precursors for Carnitine Synthesis in Human Adults," *Journal of Nutrition* 119, no. 12 (1989): 1907–13.

8. R. C. Harris, G. Jones, C. A. Hill, et al., "The Carnosine Content of V Lateralis in Vegetarians and Omnivores," abstract in *FASEB Journal* 21 (2007): 769.20.

CHAPTER 15: IS IT SAFE TO EAT SOY?

1. W. M. Rand, P. L. Pellett, and V. R. Young, "Meta-analysis of Nitrogen Balance Studies for Estimating Protein Requirements in Healthy Adults," *American Journal of Clinical Nutrition* 77 (2003): 109–27.

2. L. E. Murray-Kolb, R. Welch, E. C. Theil, and J. L. Beard, "Women with Low Iron Stores Absorb Iron from Soybeans," *American Journal of Clinical Nutrition* 77 (2003): 180–84.

3. R. P. Heaney, C. M. Weaver, and M. L. Fitzsimmons, "Soybean Phytate Content: Effect on Calcium Absorption," *American Journal of Clinical Nutrition* 53 (1991): 745–47.

4. Y. Zhao, B. R. Martin, and C. M. Weaver, "Calcium Bioavailability of Calcium Carbonate Fortified Soymilk is Equivalent to Cow's Milk in Young Women," *Journal of Nutrition* 135 (2005): 2379–82.

5. B. Lonnerdal, "Soybean Ferritin: Implications for Iron Status of Vegetarians," *American Journal of Clinical Nutrition* 89 (2009): S1680–S1685.

6. Zhao, Martin, and Weaver, "Calcium Bioavailability," 2379–82.

7. A. L. Tang, K. Z. Walker, G. Wilcox, B. J. Strauss, J. F. Ashton, and L. Stojanovska, "Calcium Absorption in Australian Osteopenic Post-menopausal Women: An Acute Comparative Study of Fortified Soymilk to Cows' Milk," *Asia Pacific Journal of Clinical Nutrition* 19 (2010): 243–49.

8. T. Oseni, R. Patel, J. Pyle, and V. C. Jordan, "Selective Estrogen Receptor Modulators and Phytoestrogens," *Planta Medica* 74 (2008): 1656–65.

9. M. Heringa, "Review on Raloxifene: Profile of a Selective Estrogen Receptor Modulator," *International Journal of Clinical Pharmacology and Therapeutics* 41 (2003): 331–45.

10. K. D. Setchell, N. M. Brown, and E. Lydeking-Olsen, "The Clinical Importance of the Metabolite Equol: A Clue to the Effectiveness of Soy and Its Isoflavones," *Journal of Nutrition* 132 (2002): 3577–84.

11. K. D. Setchell and S. J. Cole, "Method of Defining Equol-Producer Status and Its Frequency Among Vegetarians," *Journal of Nutrition* 136 (2006): 2188–93.

12. D. J. Jenkins, A. Mirrahimi, K. Srichaikul, et al., "Soy Protein Reduces Serum Cholesterol by Both Intrinsic and Food Displacement Mechanisms," *Journal of Nutrition* 140 (2010): 23025–23115.

13. Ibid.

14. M. S. Rosell, P. N. Appleby, E. A. Spencer, and T. J. Key, "Soy Intake and Blood Cholesterol Concentrations: A Cross-sectional Study of 1033 Pre- and Postmenopausal Women in the Oxford Arm of the European Prospective Investigation into Cancer and Nutrition," *American Journal of Clinical Nutrition* 80 (2004): 1391–96.

15. C. Nagata, N. Takatsuka, Y. Kurisu, and H. Shimizu, "Decreased Serum Total Cholesterol Concentration is Associated with High Intake of Soy Products in Japanese Men and Women," *Journal of Nutrition* 128 (1998): 209–13.

16. M. R. Law, N. J. Wald, and S. G. Thompson, "By How Much and How Quickly Does Reduction in Serum Cholesterol Concentration Lower Risk of Ischaemic Heart Disease?" *British Medical Journal* 308 (1994): 367–72.

17. M. R. Law, N. J. Wald, T. Wu, A. Hackshaw, and A. Bailey, "Systematic Underestimation of Association between Serum Cholesterol Concentration and Ischaemic Heart Disease in Observational Studies: Data from the BUPA Study," *British Medical Journal* 308 (1994): 363–66.

18. D. J. Jenkins, C. W. Kendall, D. Faulkner, et al., "A Dietary Portfolio Approach to Cholesterol Reduction: Combined Effects of Plant Sterols, Vegetable Proteins, and Viscous Fibers in Hypercholesterolemia," *Metabolism* 51 (2002): 1596–604.

19. S. Desroches, J. F. Mauger, L. M. Ausman, A. H. Lichtenstein, and B. Lamarche, "Soy Protein Favorably Affects LDL Size Independently of Isoflavones in Hypercholesterolemic Men and Women. *Journal of Nutrition* 134 (2004): 574–79.

20. X. Zhang, X. O. Shu, Y. T. Gao, et al., "Soy Food Consumption is Associated with Lower Risk of Coronary Heart Disease in Chinese Women," *Journal of Nutrition* 133 (2003): 2874–78.

21. S. Sasazuki, "Case-Control Study of Nonfatal Myocardial Infarction in Relation to Selected Foods in Japanese Men and Women," *Japanese Circulation Journal* 65 (2001): 200–06.

22. Y. Kokubo, H. Iso, J. Ishihara, K. Okada, M. Inoue, and S. Tsugane, "Association of Dietary Intake of Soy, Beans, and Isoflavones with Risk of Cerebral and Myocardial Infarctions in Japanese Populations: The Japan Public Health Center-based (JPHC) Study Cohort I," *Circulation* 116 (2007): 2553–62.

23. W. Liang, A. H. Lee, C. W. Binns, R. Huang, D. Hu, and H. Shao, "Soy Consumption Reduces Risk of Ischemic Stroke: A Case-Control Study in Southern China," *Neuroepidemiology* 33 (2009): 111–16.

24. S. H. Li, X. X. Liu, Y. Y. Bai, et al., "Effect of Oral Isoflavone Supplementation on Vascular Endothelial Function in Postmenopausal Women: A Meta-analysis of Randomized Placebo-Controlled Trials," *American Journal of Clinical Nutrition* 91 (2010): 480–86.

25. Writing Group for the Women's Health Initiative Investigators, "Risks and Benefits of Estrogen Plus Progestin in Healthy Postmenopausal Women: Principal Results from the Women's Health Initiative Randomized Controlled Trial," *Journal of the American Medical Association* 288 (2002): 321–33.

26. D. F. Ma, L. Q. Qin, P. Y. Wang, and R. Katoh, "Soy Isoflavone Intake Increases Bone Mineral Density in the Spine of Menopausal Women: Meta-analysis of Randomized Controlled Trials," *Clinical Nutrition* 27 (2008): 57–64.

27. K. Taku, M. K. Melby, J. Takebayashi, et al., "Effect of Soy Isoflavone Extract Supplements on Bone Mineral Density in Menopausal Women: Meta-analysis of Randomized Controlled Trials," *Asia Pacific Journal of Clinical Nutrition* 19 (2010): 33–42.

28. J. Liu, S. C. Ho, Y. X. Su, W. Q. Chen, C. X. Zhang, and Y. M. Chen, "Effect of Long-term Intervention of Soy Isoflavones on Bone Mineral Density in Women: A Meta-analysis of Randomized Controlled Trials," *Bone* 44 (2009): 948–53.

29. W. P. Koh, A. H. Wu, R. Wang, et al., "Gender-Specific Associations between Soy and Risk of Hip Fracture in the Singapore Chinese Health Study," *American Journal of Epidemiology* 170 (2009): 901–09.

30. X. Zhang, X. O. Shu, H. Li, et al., "Prospective Cohort Study of Soy Food Consumption and Risk of Bone Fracture among Postmenopausal Women," *Archives of Internal Medicine* 165 (2005): 1890–95.

31. R. Bolanos, A. D. Castillo, and J. Francia, "Soy Isoflavones versus Placebo in the Treatment of Climacteric Vasomotor Symptoms: Systematic Review and Meta-analysis," *Menopause: The Journal of the North American Menopause Society* 17 (2010): 1–7.

32. H. D. Nelson, K. K. Vesco, E. Haney, et al., "Nonhormonal Therapies for Menopausal Hot Flashes: Systematic Review and Meta-analysis," *Journal of the American Medical Association* 295 (2006): 2057–71.

33. L. G. Howes, J. B. Howes, and D. C. Knight, "Isoflavone Therapy for Menopausal Flushes: A Systematic Review and Meta-analysis," *Maturitas* 55 (2006): 203–11.

34. H. Wiseman, K. Casey, E. A. Bowey, et al., "Influence of 10 Weeks of Soy Consumption on Plasma Concentrations and Excretion of Isoflavonoids and on Gut Microflora Metabolism in Healthy Adults," *American Journal of Clinical Nutrition* 80 (2004): 692–99.

35. M. Messina and S. Barnes, "The Role of Soy Products in Reducing Risk of Cancer," *Journal of the National Cancer Institute* 83 (1991): 541–46.

36. Y. Folman and G. S. Pope, "The Interaction in the Immature Mouse of Potent Oestrogens with Coumestrol, Genistein and Other Utero-vaginotrophic Compounds of Low Potency," *Journal of Endocrinology* 34 (1966): 215–25.

37. Y. Folman and G. S. Pope, "Effect of Norethisterone Acetate, Dimethyl-stilboestrol, Genistein and Coumestrol on Uptake of [3H]oestradiol by Uterus, Vagina and Skeletal Muscle of Immature Mice," *Journal of Endocrinology* 44 (1969): 213–18.

38. P. Pisani, F. Bray, and D. M. Parkin, "Estimates of the Worldwide Prevalence of Cancer for 25 Sites in the Adult Population," *International Journal of Cancer* 97 (2002): 72–81.

39. W. G. Helferich, J. E. Andrade, and M. S. Hoagland, "Phytoestrogens and Breast Cancer: A Complex Story," *Inflammopharmacology* 16 (2008): 219–26.

40. C. D. Allred, K. F. Allred, Y. H. Ju, T. S. Goeppinger, D. R. Doerge, and W. G. Helferich, "Soy Processing Influences Growth of Estrogen-Dependent Breast Cancer Tumors," *Carcinogenesis* 25 (2004): 1649–57.

41. M. Messina, D. I. Abrams, and M. Hardy, "Can Clinicians Now Assure Their Breast Cancer Patients That Soyfoods Are Safe?" *Womens Health* 6 (2010): 335–38.

42. C. Doyle, L. H. Kushi, T. Byers, et al., "Nutrition and Physical Activity During and After Cancer Treatment: An American Cancer Society Guide for Informed Choices," *CA: A Cancer Journal for Clinicians* 56 (2006): 323–53.

43. X. O. Shu, Y. Zheng, H. Cai, et al., "Soy Food Intake and Breast Cancer Survival," *JAMA* 302 (2009): 2437–43.

44. X. Kang, Q. Zhang, S. Wang, X. Huang, and S. Jin, "Effect of Soy Isoflavones on Breast Cancer Recurrence and Death for Patients Receiving Adjuvant Endocrine Therapy," *Canadian Medical Association Journal* 182 (2010): 1821.

45. M. Messina and A. H. Wu, "Perspectives on the Soy-Breast Cancer Relation," *American Journal of Clinical Nutrition* 89 (2009): S1673–S1679.

46. M. Messina and L. Hilakivi-Clarke, "Early Intake Appears to Be the Key to the Proposed Protective Effects of Soy Intake Against Breast Cancer," *Nutrition and Cancer* 61 (2009): 792–98.

47. Pisani, Bray, and Parkin, "Estimates of the Worldwide Prevalence of Cancer for 25 Sites in the Adult Population," 72–81.

48. L. Yan and E. L. Spitznagel, "Soy Consumption and Prostate Cancer Risk in Men: A Revisit of a Meta-analysis," *American Journal of Clinical Nutrition* 89 (2009): 1155–63.

49. L. Xu, Y. Ding, W. J. Catalona, et al., "MEK4 Function, Genistein Treatment, and Invasion of Human Prostate Cancer Cells," *Journal of the National Cancer Institute* 101 (2009): 1141–55.

50. L. R. White, H. Petrovitch, G. W. Ross, et al., "Brain Aging and Midlife Tofu Consumption," *Journal of the American College of Nutrition* 19 (2000): 242–55.

51. Ibid.

52. J. Woo, H. Lynn, W. Y. Lau, et al., "Nutrient Intake and Psychological Health in an Elderly Chinese Population," *International Journal of Geriatric Psychiatry* 21 (2006): 1036–43.

53. L. Zhao and R. D. Brinton, "WHI and WHIMS Follow-up and Human Studies of Soy Isoflavones on Cognition," *Expert Review of Neurotherapeutics* 7 (2007): 1549–64.

54. D. R. Doerge and D. M. Sheehan, "Goitrogenic and Estrogenic Activity of Soy Isoflavones," *Environmental Health Perspective* 110, suppl. no. 3 (2002): 349–53.

55. M. Messina and G. Redmond, "Effects of Soy Protein and Soybean Isoflavones on Thyroid Function in Healthy Adults and Hypothyroid Patients: A Review of the Relevant Literature," *Thyroid* 16 (2006): 249–58.

56. A. Bitto, F. Polito, M. Atteritano, et al., "Genistein Aglycone Does Not Affect Thyroid Function: Results from a Three-Year, Randomized, Double-Blind, Placebo-Controlled Trial," *Journal of Clinical Endocrinology and Metabolism* 95 (2010): 3067–72.

57. J. M. Hamilton-Reeves, G. Vazquez, S. J. Duval, W. R. Phipps, M. S. Kurzer, and M. J. Messina, "Clinical Studies Show No Effects of Soy Protein or Isoflavones on Reproductive Hormones in Men: Results of a Meta-analysis," *Fertility and Sterility* 94 (2010): 997–1007.

58. M. Messina, "Soybean Isoflavone Exposure Does Not Have Feminizing Effects on Men: A Critical Examination of the Clinical Evidence," *Fertility and Sterility* 93 (2010): 2095–2104.

59. J. E. Chavarro, T. L. Toth, S. M. Sadio, and R. Hauser, "Soy Food and Isoflavone Intake in Relation to Semen Quality Parameters Among Men from an Infertility Clinic," *Human Reproduction* 23 (2008): 2584–90.

60. M. Messina, "Soybean Isoflavone Exposure Does Not Have Feminizing Effects on Men," 2095–2104.

61. M. L. Casini, S. Gerli, and V. Unfer, "An Infertile Couple Suffering from Oligospermia by Partial Sperm Maturation Arrest: Can Phytoestrogens Play a Therapeutic Role? A Case Report Study," *Gynecological Endocrinology* 22 (2006): 399–401.

62. M. Messina, C. Nagata, and A. H. Wu, "Estimated Asian Adult Soy Protein and Isoflavone Intakes," *Nutrition and Cancer* 55 (2006): 1–12.

63. Rand, Pellett, and Young, "Meta-analysis of Nitrogen Balance Studies," 109–27.

64. M. Messina, Nagata, and Wu, "Estimated Asian Adult Soy Protein and Isoflavone Intakes," 1–12.

CHAPTER 16: WHY VEGAN?

1. PETA investigation of Aviagen Turkeys Inc.: http://www.peta.org/mc/NewsItem.asp?id=12245.

2. Ian Duncan, "Animal Welfare Issues in the Poultry Industry: Is There a Lesson to Be Learned?" *Journal of Applied Animal Welfare Science* 4, no. 3 (2001): 207–21.

3. A. B. Webster, "Welfare Implications of Avian Osteoporosis," *Poultry Science* 83 (2004): 184–92.

4. Compassion Over Killing investigation of Michael Foods: http://www.cok .net/inthenews/releases/?pr=dunkincruelty-farm-investigation.

5. Mercy For Animals investigation of Quality Eggs: http://www.mercyfor animals.org/maine-eggs/.

6. Mercy For Animals investigation of Norco Ranch: http://www.upc-online .org/battery_hens/101608norco.html.

7. Duncan, "Animal Welfare Issues in the Poultry Industry," 207–21.

8. L. A. Gustafson, H. W. Cheng, J. P. Garner, E. A. Pajor, and J. A. Mench, "The Effects of Different Bill-Trimming Methods," *Poultry Science* 86 (2007): 1831–39.

9. Duncan, "Animal Welfare Issues in the Poultry Industry," 207–21.

10. PETA investigation of Aviagen Turkeys Inc.: http://www.peta.org/mc/ NewsItem.asp?id=12245.

11. Duncan, "Animal Welfare Issues in the Poultry Industry," 207–21.

12. Compassion Over Killing investigation of Hudson Valley Foie Gras: http://www.cok.net/feat/hudsonvalley.php.

13. E. A. Pajor, "Group Housing of Sows in Small Pens: Advantages, Disadvantages and Recent Research," in *Proceedings: Symposium on Sow Housing and Well-being*, Des Moines, IA, June 5, 2002, ces.purdue.edu/pork/sowhousing/ swine_02.pdf.

14. Highlights of Swine 2006 Part III: Reference of Swine Health, Productivity, and General Management in the United States, 2006, Animal and Plant Health Inspection Service, USDA, March 2008, http://www.aphis.usda.gov/animal _health/nahms/swine/index.shtml.

15. Ibid.

16. PETA investigation of Murphy Family Ventures: http://www.foxnews .com/story/0,2933,316624,00.html.

17. PETA investigation of Hormel: http://www.peta.org/b/thepetafiles/archive/ 2008/10/22/22-charges-filed-based-on-peta-investigation-at-hormel-supplier .aspx.

18. Mercy For Animals investigation of Country View Family Farms: http://www .mercyforanimals.org/pigs/.

19. USDA National Agricultural Statistics Service Quick Stats: http://www .nass.usda.gov/QuickStats.

20. PETA investigation of Land O'Lakes: https://secure.peta.org/site/Advocacy?cmd=display&page=UserAction&id=2515.

21. Mercy For Animals investigation of Willet Dairy: http://www.mercyforanimals.org/dairy/.

22. Humane Society of the United States Report: "The Welfare of Animals in the Veal Industry," September 5, 2008, http://www.humanesociety.org/assets/pdfs/farm/hsus-the-welfare-of-animals-in-the-veal-industry.pdf (accessed November 11, 2009).

23. Ibid.

24. Humane Society of the United States, "HSUS Investigation Results in Closure of Vermont Slaughter Plant," October 30, 2009, http://www.humanesociety.org/news/press_releases/2009/10/vt_slaughter_plant_investigation_103009.html.

25. Compassion Over Killing investigation of transport of animals: http://www.cok.net/feat/usti.php.

26. Temple Grandin, "Recommended Captive Bolt Stunning Techniques for Cattle, www.grandin.com/humane/cap.bolt.tips.html (accessed October 28, 2009).

27. Kurt Vogel and Temple Grandin, "2008 Restaurant Animal Welfare and Humane Slaughter Audits in Federally Inspected Beef and Pork Slaughter Plants in the U.S. and Canada," http://www.grandin.com/survey/2008.restaurant.audits.html (accessed October 28, 2009); and Livestock Slaughter 2008 Summary, United States Department of Agriculture: Economics, Statistics, and Market Information System, http://usda.mannlib.cornell.edu/usda/nass/LiveSlauSu//2000s/2009/LiveSlauSu-03-06-2009.pdf.

28. Grandin, "Recommended Captive Bolt Stunning Techniques for Cattle," www.grandin.com/humane/cap.bolt.tips.html.

29. Joby Warrik, "Modern Meat: A Brutal Harvest," *Washington Post*, April 10, 2001.

30. Jean-Pierre Ruiz, "USDA Veterinarian Testifies Agency Endangers Public Health," *Seattle Examiner*, March 5, 2010, http://www.examiner.com/x-9726-Seattle-Pet-Laws-Examiner~y2010m3d6-Veterinarian-calls-for-overhaul-of-USDA-slaughterhouse-rules.

31. USDA Poultry Slaughter 2008 Annual Summary, http://usda.mannlib.cornell.edu/usda/nass/PoulSlauSu//2000s/2009/PoulSlauSu-02-25-2009.pdf.

32. PETA investigation of Tyson Foods 2004–2005: https://secure.peta.org/site/Advocacy?cmd=display&page=UserAction&id=1121.

33. PETA investigation of Tyson Foods 2008: http://www.northcountrygazette.org/2008/01/18/peta-accuses-tyson-of-chicken-abuse/.

34. Mercy For Animals investigation of House of Raeford Farms: http://newsblaze.com/story/20070601091318rose.nb/topstory.html.

35. Temple Grandin, "Electric Stunning of Pigs and Sheep," updated June 2008, http://www.grandin.com/humane/elec.stun.html.

36. Ben Harris, "PETA Says Agriprocessors Misled Rabbis About Slaughter Procedures," http://www.jewishjournal.com/food/article/peta_says_agriprocessors_misled_rabbis_about_slaughter_procedures_video_200/.

37. Andy Coghlan, "Animals Feel the Pain of Religious Slaughter," NewScientist, October 13, 2009, http://www.newscientist.com/article/dn17972-animals-feel-the-pain-of-religious-slaughter.html?DCMP=OTC-rss&nsref=online-news (accessed October 15, 2009).

38. "If This is Kosher . . . " narrated by Jonathan Safran Foer, http://video.google.com/videoplay?docid=-7330038074290819722#.

39. Feedstuffs on Factory Farm Cruelties, Vegan.com, September 28, 2009, http://www.vegan.com/blog/2009/09/28/feedstuffs-on-factory-farm-cruelties/.

INDEX